Finding Your Feet

How the Sole reflects the Soul

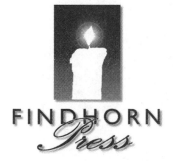

FINDHORN
Press

Finding Your Feet

How the Sole reflects the Soul

Ann Gadd

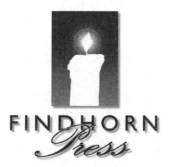

FINDHORN
Press

First published in English by Findhorn Press 2006

ISBN 10: 1-84409-081-7
ISBN 13: 978-1-84409-081-5

British Library Cataloguing-in-Publication Data.
A catalogue record for this book is available
from the British Library.

Edited by Jane Engel
Illustrations by Anthony Gadd
Cover and interior design by Damian Keenan
Printed and bound by WS Bookwell, Finland

1 2 3 4 5 6 7 8 9 10 11 12 13 12 11 10 09 08 07 06

Published by
Findhorn Press
305a The Park, Findhorn
Forres IV36 3TE
Scotland, UK

Telephone
01309 - 690582
Fax
01309 - 690036

info@findhornpress.com
www.findhornpress.com

CONTENTS

Introduction

SECTION I

SECTION II

Dedication

To all the very special souls whose sole stories have made this book possible, my huge love and thanks as without you this would not have been possible; to the most precious souls with whom I share my life, especially Anthony, Tess, Taun and my furry friends; to Brenda whom I'm so fortunate to have as a guide; to Lydia who read the book first; to Chris Stormer for finding the original path, Jenny for the beach walks; Nicky Eastment for the legal issues, and all those of you who cared. Thank you.

Acknowledgments

*Findhorn Press for seeing the potential, Anthony who did the illustrations so well and efficiently, my children, Tess and Taun, Stan and Ruth, brother Gareth and sister Glynis, friends, especially Annette, Anthea, Gillian, Jane, Jeanine, Jenny(s), Jos, Lydia, Marianne, Marleen, Marriette, Mel(s), Shelly, Sheleen and Val.
You're what make life
so special.*

Feet First

"This is the truth, the whole truth and nothing but the truth: As below, so above; and as above, so below. With this knowledge alone you may work miracles." **Hermes Trismegistos.** [1]

"In one atom are found all the elements of the earth; in one motion of the mind are found the motions of all the laws of existence; in one drop of water are found the secrets of all the endless oceans; in one aspect of you are found all the aspects of existence." **Kahlil Gibran.** [2]

We walk on them, we use them to kick, to run, to dangle, to play footsie-footsie, to stand on and to move through life. We dress them in expensive footwear and get sensual pleasure strolling barefoot on soft grass with them. Yet we often find them unacceptable, either because of their shape or odor. Relegated to the lowest position on our physical self, for the most part we ignore them – our feet.

Each foot has 26 bones, more than 100 ligaments and 19 muscles. The feet work very hard – during the course of a single day they are subjected to weight loads equivalent to several hundred tons. Yet in spite of their underdog position, the feet have a profound gift of insight to give to each of us, as you'll discover when you explore their symbolic potential. From warts to bunions, nothing occurs on our feet by chance. As such, they reflect our innermost selves.

The relevance of the feet to our emotional selves, was known by past civilizations, mystics and seers, but was largely dismissed as nonsense with the advent of allopathic medicine. Yet gradually this information that has previously remained hidden is coming to light and is being more widely accepted.

The idea that our feet could be a mirror for the path we have and are walking through life, could be viewed to be absurd, - some weird flight of sensational fancy. No more so though, than having needles stuck into our ears to cure sinusitis, as in acupuncture; or taking the essence of a disease and diluting it to such an extent as to leave a minute fraction of the original essence. So logic would decree that it could have no effect at all (particularly when we discover the more the original essence is diluted, the greater its strength becomes). Yet homeopathy works on just this principal the more subtle an essence, the greater its effect on the gross or physical body. Iridology works on the principal that the eyes reflect the body, just as crystallization-testing does with drops of our blood. (Blood crystallization is a procedure whereby a sample of blood is left to dry on a glass slide. It is then examined and based on the appearance of the coagulated blood, microscopists are able to determine – by examining the clots of protein puddles in the blood - whether there are inflammatory or degenerative problems.) Human genetics works on the same principal, which Kahlil Gibran alludes to when he says that a single atom contains all the earth's elements. There are many more examples of this and there are even allopathic medicine practitioners who understand that a part of the body is representative of the whole.

In psycho-immunology, contemporary medicine realizes that there is a link between a patient's emotional state and his or her physical well-being and that what happens to one will reflect in the other and in light of this, the premise that our soles reflect our souls, becomes possible.

I have worked for over 15 years assisting people, through counseling, Reiki and other techniques, to discover their behavioural patterns and release those that they feel do not serve them. The majority of people who come to see me do not have major physical diseases yet almost all have emotional problems. Psychotherapy, while highly recommended, is often a lengthy and expensive process which excludes many people from enjoying its benefits. Consequently, I looked for another tool that could bring us to a deeper understanding of ourselves and enrich our lives before our bodies became ill. This book then serves as a beginner's guide to understanding the feet. I have provided case histories to best illustrate the individual aspects of the feet and to make their occurrence more understandable.

My search led me to study the relationship between behavioural patterns and different food characteristics. Up till then much of what I intuitively diagnosed was based on the client resonating and accepting what I said. This is, in some respects, a disempowering process in that clients have to rely on the healer's insights to assist them, as opposed to getting information and drawing their own conclusions. However, through understanding our habits or examining our feet, we can draw our own insights.

Many times letting go of past unbalancing issues comes through the acceptance and understanding of their cause. Having discovered and resonating with possible causes, it is then up to us to decide if we want to make the relevant changes.

In summary then the aim of the book is to:

- allow us to become more conscious of ourselves and others
- empower us to assume responsibility for our own healing
- release and make changes we feel appropriate

I first came to understand the relevance of my feet when I left my exciting career in advertising to have children. Leaving my job was very hard to do, as I had thrived on the prestige and power it afforded me and it was hard to replace the boardroom drama with nappies. I found the change quite traumatic and missed the company of my colleagues. Somehow, much as I adored her, my screaming wet bundle did not offer the same stimulation. I was lonely, depressed and not sure how to cope with motherhood that offered no step-by-step manual. At that time, the soles of my feet peeled completely. It was as if the new role I was stepping into, literally involved *shedding skin*, as the old disintegrated to make way for the very different life awaiting me. Then, my toes were bent to the point that the nails on all but the big toe were not visible from the top. As I began to explore not only my procreative but creative potential, by painting and writing, so the toes gradually unfurled and my shoe size went from a six and a half to an eight.

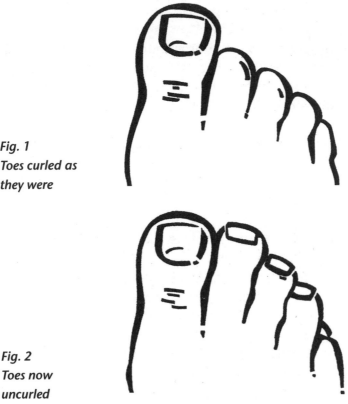

Fig. 1
Toes curled as
they were

Fig. 2
Toes now
uncurled

Chris Stormer's book, *The Language of the Feet*,[1] helped me to under-stand the changes and nuances of the feet. As the feet represent each aspect of the body, by working with them Reflexologists work with the entire body, however in this book I have focused on ailments and fea-tures that specifically affect the feet.

When I look at someone's feet, I often feel as if I am talking to an old person who is full of stories that are just waiting to be told. Parts of the feet literally seem to light up to attract attention. Pay too much attention to one foot and the other demands attention too. Often, after the story has been heard and the emotions that accompany their telling are released, the feature that attracted my attention clears or alters, so that before, during and after a session, the feet may have altered considerably, in colour, texture, weight and lines. This never ceases to fill me with awe, and constantly reminds me of the words *"as above so below."*

For example, one person I saw, a doctor, had a very obvious line across the heel pad of her foot where the sciatic nerve is located. When I asked her about this, she mentioned having problems in this area, resulting in a shortening of her body height, as well as lower back and

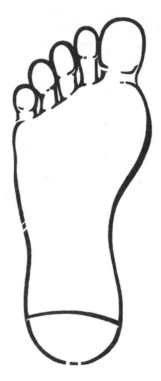

Fig. 3
Sciatica

pelvic pains. We spoke at length about various emotional issues that may have resulted in this damage. Then she had a short Reiki treatment. The long indent on both feet was so pronounced, that the following day I asked if she would mind if I could photograph them for this book, as it was such a clear example of the sciatic nerve. She agreed; however when I went to take the photo, the deep wrinkle-type indent had completely disappeared on both feet. Momentary frustration at the ruined photo opportunity, gave way to a profound sense of wonder at the healing that can take place when we have the chance to express what we have repressed.

However, we cannot always rely on others, because of location, time or finance, to sift through our lives, to unearth the hidden aspects of ourselves and reveal to the light that which was held in the shadowy darkness of our past. This book is a guide, for you the reader, to be able to work with your feet and allow them to reveal to you that which needs healing. The understanding, acceptance and forgiveness of past issues may be all that is required for you to heal. However, if the issue remains, then you may need the help of a counselor, psychologist or another professional to assist you through the process. Having identified where your problem may lie, you can facilitate this process. By learning to understand the markings on your feet, you will have an easy access guide for self-evolvement.

It's a bit like the analogy of a car running out of petrol. One may keep fixing the symptom, by going to the garage and filling up, but avoid finding the cause which may be a hole in the petrol tank. No amount of petrol is ever going to fix the hole. It will simply cost a lot of money and frustration and many unforeseen stops at the side of the road. We are often too concerned with the symptom and far less concerned with the underlying cause.

While I fully acknowledge that there are certain physical factors, such as incorrect shoes, accidents, fungal infections etc that contribute to various aspects of what occurs on our feet, I do not believe these to be the only causal factors for what transpires. For too long we have claimed to be innocent of what manifests in our bodies and have failed to grasp the rich symbology that understanding the psychological aspects of our ailments offers. I hope this book will assist you further on this path of discovery.

(Please note when examining the feet one sees various aspects in totality. However for the sake of demonstrating case histories, I have for the most part, isolated specific issues. I have also changed names and certain details of people which, while not affecting the content, provide them protection and privacy. We each have our own issues to work with in life and their stories can assist us in gaining greater understanding of our own emotions, as opposed to being in any way judgmental of theirs.

I have used case histories because I have found that we remember stories long after we have forgotten reams of factual information. Also you may well be able to identify with the people whose stories are told, or to see similarities of your own or with your patients, which will assist you.

NOTE: *When I work with someone, I create a broad scenario into which the client fills in the specific details, in response to questions. Then the condensed answers make up the case histories given.*

Where emotional issues arise as a result of insights with yourself or others, it may be wise to seek the support of a trained therapist to help you (or them) work through these issues.

This book is not intended to be a tool for physical diagnosis – I leave that to the relevant allopathic practitioners. I have tried though to be as accurate as possible about the physical causes of various ailments; however in some cases medical opinion does conflict, vary or differ widely, making the task of creating an overview difficult. Please always consult your medical practitioner for his/her view.

Once again, a huge thanks to all those people who agreed to have me include their histories and their generous contributions to this book.

SECTION 1

CHAPTER 1

From Fibonacci to Feet
Why our soles reflect our souls

How could our feet be mirrors of our souls?

To answer this question and to understand the possibility that our bodies are mirrored on our feet, we need to go back in time to 1175AD, when a man called Leonardo Pisano was born in Pisa, Italy. Leonardo, or Fibonacci as he was nicknamed, travelled widely around the Mediterranean region while working for his father's export business. During his travels, he encountered the Moors (the Muslim people living in North Africa), who taught him the Hindu-Arabic number system of 0123456789 and its decimal point. Until then, the Roman numerical system was used throughout Europe (1, 11, 111, 1V, V, V1, V11, V111, 1X, X etc). Fibonacci introduced this new system into the Western world, which we still use today.

Surprisingly though, the introduction of our numerical system, is not what Fibonacci has become famous for; rather it is a string of numbers called the "Fibonacci Series" which propelled him into the historic limelight. And, it's this system that - is useful in terms of answering our original question, how could our feet be mirrors of our souls?

It started when he posed the following question to himself:
What would happen if a pair of rabbits took a month to reach maturity, and a month to gestate, and then give birth to a pair of rabbits who would do likewise? How many rabbits would be produced over time?

The answer is as follows:

Beginning.	**- 1 pair**
At the end of the first month the rabbits are mature enough to mate.	**- 1 pair**
At the end of the second month they produce a new pair	**- 2 pairs**
At the end of the third month the original pair produces a second pair.	**- 3 pairs**
By the end of the fourth month the original pair has produced a third pair, and this new pair produces their first pair, making in total	**- 5 pairs**

If you continue with this example you will see the number of pairs growing as follows:

1, 1, 2, 3, 5, 8, 13, 21, 34, 55, 89, 144, 233, 377...

It was this sequence of numbers that got Fibonacci excited.

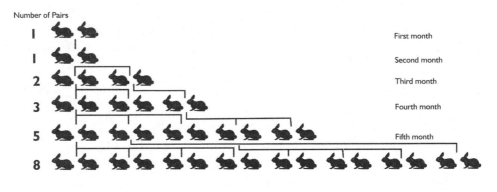

Fig. 4 Breeding Bunnies

Busy Bunnies! Not too profound you might think, except that on closer examination, there is an interesting pattern to these numbers.

The pattern is as follows: if we add together any of the two preceding numbers of the series, the first two numbers will amount to the number in front, i.e. 1 + 1 = 2, or 8 + 13 =21. This series of numbers is known as the Fibonacci sequence. If you divide each number by the number before it and, starting from one the results will look like this: 1, 2, 1.5, 1.666..., 1.6, 1.625, 1.61538, 1.619, 1.618, 1.618, 1.618 etc. As you can see, from 233 divided by 144, the result levels out at the ratio of 1.618, which is known as the Golden Mean or Golden Section.

It is represented by the Greek letter Phi or phi, as you may have learnt it at school, namely .618034.

If we examine the world around us, we will see that this ratio is reflected in many, many aspects of nature. For instance, the ratio of male bees to female bees in a hive is 1: 618. The number of petals on plants frequently are 3, 5, 8 etc. On our bodies, if you take the distance from the feet to the belly button and from the belly button to the top of the head, the ratio of these two measurements (in the average person will be 1: 618). From the tip of the hand to the elbow and from the elbow to the shoulder produces the same ratio. The fingers also reflect phi. Just look at the ratio of the middle finger's longest bone to the middle bone and the middle to the shortest bone. In fact, this ratio is found throughout our body parts. Shells correspond to this ratio (see illustration), as does Beethoven's *Moonlight Sonata*; also most business cards conform to this ratio, as do certain pure bred dogs, Notre Dame Cathedral and countless other objects.

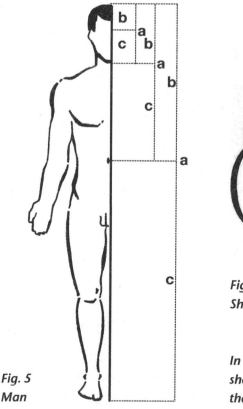

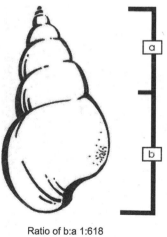

Ratio of b:a 1:618

Fig. 6
Shell

Fig. 5
Man

In these pictures of the shell and the man, the ratio of c:b is 1: 618.

In practically all Mozart's sonatas, we find a divide into sections exactly as in the Golden Section proportion. He was known to be fascinated with numbers and so this mirror of the Golden Section was undoubtedly planned and not co-incidental. By composing music according to the perfect balance, Mozart's music brings the listener into harmonious balance as well.

Knowing then that Mozart's music is harmonious to the Golden Mean, it is easy to see that through this balance mechanism, the emotions are brought into balance when the music is played. Mozart's music is not the only music that has this effect, but because it was written with the Golden Mean ratio in mind, it consciously exploits the balance principle.

This Golden Mean is also found on the foot as shown in the diagram below, where the distance from the heel to the ball of the foot and from the ball of the foot to the tips of the toes is, on an average foot, in the ratio 1:618. Likewise the distance from the ball of the foot to the neck of the toes and tips of toes, and from the necks of the toes to the toe pads, and toes pads to tips of the toes are also usually in the ratio 1:618.

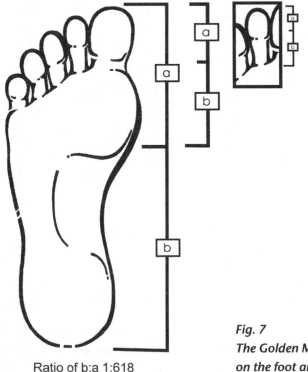

Ratio of b:a 1:618

Fig. 7
The Golden Mean
on the foot and toes

Taking this configuration of numbers further, and translating the dimensions into squares as shown in the diagram, we can create a spiral that also correlates to many other things found in the universe.

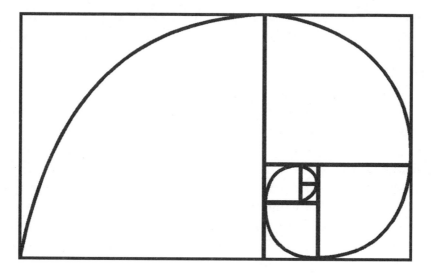

*Fig. 8 · **The Golden Mean translated into a spiral***

This shape and its mathematical principals, known as the Golden Mean, are reflected in many aspects of creation, from architecture, classical art, the formation of galaxies to the head of a cauliflower!

There are many other aspects of our world that repeat themselves patterns that, if studied, can be used to give us insights into our lives. Understanding the correlations in our lives through divination, allows us to connect the dots or gain insight. Then, being more aware, hopefully we don't repeat these patterns, but rather create new ones. In doing so we become more integrated, or whole, which translates spiritually, as holy. We speak of the great divide – the illusion that we are separate. Understanding these divine patterns or connections such as the Golden Mean, allows us to experience that we aren't separate; that no matter how insignificant we believe ourselves to be, we are nevertheless part of something far greater. Much of our growth in life relates to understanding our patterns, and becoming aware of our actions and emotions, which we can do in any number of ways, from reading teacups, to astrology, or observing our feet. Then we can understand that, like the Golden Mean, these patterns which we now are aware of can be recognized in other areas of life.

"However high a state the soul may have attained, self-knowledge is incumbent upon it, and this it will never be able to neglect even if it should so desire." **St. Teresa of Avila.** [1]

The reason divination works (for instance in studying the aspects of the feet) is because these patterns show us the interrelatedness of all that is.

Divination

Divination has been used by man from the earliest of times and was in many instances essential for survival, such as using a divining, or dowsing rod to find for water, or divining for information as to where game was to be located before a hunt. There are literally thousands of divining tools, from the *I Ching*, to numerology, hand-writing analysis, astrology, palmistry to the ancient African Hakata, (which involves throwing three pieces of flat wood with different markings to get answers). Pythagoras, the Greek mathematician was known to use the flight of birds as a divination tool.

The word divination relates to the word 'divine' or God. So through divining, we utilize the concept that all is one, or that God (or the divine) is reflected in all that is. The macrocosm reflects the microcosm and vice versa or put differently, all things are related to every other thing. By studying the formation of an atom then we can relate this information to the formation of the galaxies. For example, we will find that the percentage difference between the positions of the planets in the galaxy, is the same as the percentage difference between the protons and neutrons in an atom. By studying one we learn more about the other. This principle of relating things is the core reason why divination tools work.

Science has proven that electrons and photons respond according to statistical laws i.e. their movement is not random. We also know that when an atom is split by changing one particle from negative to positive, this causes a reversal in the charge to the other part, even when they are separated. Thus we can prove their connection, and in turn the connection between all things.

When something is described as separate it means that things or people are no longer in communication or contact and so cannot affect each other. However science has shown us that the smallest building blocks of matter are in some way connected and share information.

Using the principal of the microcosm mirroring the macrocosm, it's only logical then to assume that this connectedness exists amongst all things.

So nothing happens without a reason, or put another way, anything that occurs impacts on the individual and in turn the rest of humanity.

What relevance is this then to your feet?

Simply this – in this incredible universe there are patterns that repeat themselves, as reflected in the quote from the Lord's Prayer, *"on earth as it is in heaven."* From the DNA structure of the molecules of our body, to a spiraling galaxy, there is a divine pattern or cosmic brush-stroke in our world. Through divination, no matter what tool we use, we simply interpret these patterns.

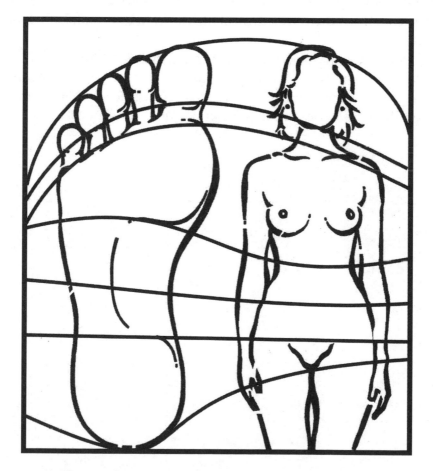

Fig. 9 · An illustration to indicate how the body fits on the sole

Therefore, it is not only possible, but also probable, that our entire bodies are reflected in other parts of our bodies such as our heads, hands and feet. These smaller parts then, become the microcosm of the macrocosm that is our body. The hands in palmistry mirror the body, as does the head (a principle used in Indian head massage), while Reflexology works on the same principle using the feet. With this in mind, then it becomes possible to believe that all aspects of our physical, emotional, mental and spiritual bodies are represented on our feet. More simply put, our souls mirror our soles.

Why would one choose understanding the feet as opposed to other divinatory tools? Simply because we always carry our feet with us; they are very visible and consequently easy to examine and have aspects that are very apparent. It's also a non-invasive way of understanding someone you may be working with and is particularly useful when working with children, who are not always able to verbalize their emotions.

By becoming aware of our soles as more than just the bottom of our feet, we become aware of our souls and so have a tool to plumb the depths of our own being, to reach a greater degree of self-understanding, on the road to becoming more conscious.

CHAPTER 2

Soul to Sole

The seven chakras on the feet

In this chapter you will discover that it is not only the actual aspect, such as a cut or callus on the feet that is relevant to your emotional makeup, but what gives us greater insight, is *where* these or any other symptom appear. In Section Two we will examine *what* specific aspects and ailments mean, while here we are concerned with the relevance of *where* a certain aspect is located. To understand this, it is helpful to divide the foot into seven chakras, each of which relates to specific issues, starting with the heel as the first area; the lower instep as the second; the upper instep as the third; the ball of the foot as the fourth; the neck of the toes as the fifth; the lower pad as the sixth, and the top of the toe pad as the seventh area.

(Note: When you want to find out more about a wart for instance, you can go to Section Two and get information about the nature of warts, and then gain insight into specifically what areas of your life the wart reflects, by seeing in which of the seven areas of the foot it is located.)

These areas are not random. They relate to the seven main chakras or energy centres, found on the body, just as the organs, the skeletal system etc. are mirrored on the feet. These chakras form the total energetic makeup of an individual. They are vortexes of seven spinning coloured light, starting at the base of the spine and continuing up through the lower abdomen, solar plexus, heart, throat, brow and top of the head. As in the colour spectrum, red is the slowest vibrating colour and so its location is found at the base of the spine (represented on the bottom or heel of the foot) while violet vibrates the fastest and is found on the crown of the head (tops of the toes). The other colours fit in-between, mirroring a rainbow and frequently, the rainbow has been used as a metaphor for the spiritual journey. We seek the pot of gold at its end, the divine gold of enlightenment, which as in the myth, remains elusive to all but the most determined seeker.

One might assume that we know ourselves emotionally and don't need a callus to give us insight. However, it is my experience, both personally and as a holistic practitioner that while we may have acquired a degree of emotional understanding, awareness of deeper layers of our feelings for the most part either elude us or are unconscious. Therefore, we may appear to be angry but in truth the anger may be hiding a deep-rooted fear. By working with each layer of emotion, concerning a situation, we are truly able to let it go. When we release an issue, we allow ourselves to become lighter, light-hearted and more enlightened; then our life's path, however stony, becomes more understandable and tolerable. That is one of the values of becoming self-aware.

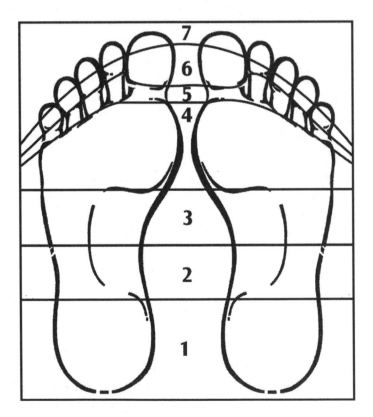

Fig. 10 · Here are the seven chakras that we divide the foot into and their related issues.

What the seven Chakras of the feet represent

Now that you understand how the foot is divided into seven chakras and you know what each chakra represents, then you can relate it to whatever aspect of the foot you can see, such as cuts, warts etc.

(Note: The toes, as well as representing chakras four, five and six horizontally (see Fig. 10) also each represent one of the first five chakras vertically, starting with the small toes representing the first chakra. So the small toe carries issues of the first chakra as well as the fifth, six and seventh chakras. This is explained in greater detail in this chapter, following the definition of the seven chakras. These vertical chakras are secondary in interpretation to the horizontal ones.

Chakra One

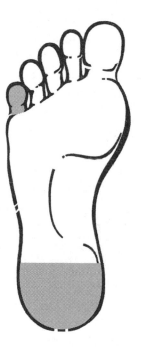

Fig. 11
First Chakra

Location of actual chakra	At the base of the spine
Location on foot	The *heel* and *small toe*
Emotional expression	Fear/anger (feeling *physically* afraid or threatened)
Relationships	To family, colleagues, race groups, religious groups and any other groups of people to whom you are affiliated

Lessons in	Trust/security/giving birth to projects/ breaking away from groups to find self and betrayal
Colour	Red
Related body parts	Anus, bowels, large intestine, legs, immune system, sciatic nerve
Key words	Fight or flight
Element	Earth

The first chakra is located on the heels of both feet. It relates to our connection to mother earth and consequently feeling rooted or connected. Someone with a large heel could consequently be well-grounded and practical. (If the heel is abnormally large it may be that the person *seeks* security and needs to ground themselves). Security issues relating to house/home would be important, whereas someone with a small or very narrow heel may be more of an etheric, airy, perhaps impractical person. For it is on the heel that issues of grounding and our tribal issues lie. If we have been inadequately nourished or constantly uprooted as a child, there may be indications of this on the right (past) heel, which could still be relevant and show up consequently on our left (present) foot. Should you have experienced this, you may have difficulties with prosperity as well as fear or anger over physical/security threats. Do you feel *well-heeled* or *down-at-heel*? Does life make you want to *take to your heels* or stand *rooted to the spot* in fright? Do you find it hard to *cool your heels?* Do you quickly get impatient with situations or people?

If our heels actually stick out behind our feet (*see Fig. 12*) then we are showing just how hard it is for us to move ahead and let go of our family/tribe. Change is hard and therefore we may want to *drag our heels.*

One client, who had been abandoned as a baby, had very small heels in comparison to the rest of her foot. Her baby toe was also very small and stood apart from the other toes. This was understandable, given her lack of roots, nurturing and bonding with her mother. Her baby toes demonstrated her feelings of isolation. The left baby toe pad also had a dark bruise, which had been there for as long as she could remember. (The left foot relates to female issues and the right foot to male issues and was a clear indication of how bruised or deeply hurt this abandonment had left her.)

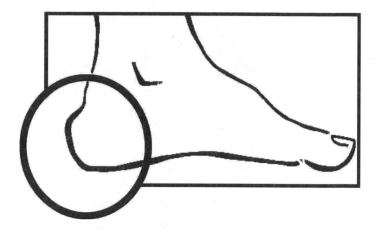

Fig. 12 · Heel showing area sticking out behind

When we feel secure, we say we have *put down roots* in a certain area. Alternatively, we establish a *home base* which relates to family, work colleagues etc. Calluses are often found on the heel, as a result of feeling the need to thicken our skin (*thick skinned* as in not wanting to be sensitive to something or someone) in order to feel less vulnerable, either as a result of security or family/work related issues. Having our security threatened, may make us feel vulnerable, as in our *Achilles' heel.*

A situation or person may also make us *feel like a heel,* i.e. someone in the lowest position. On the other hand, we may *dig our heels in,* when we stubbornly refuse to budge.

Ask someone to feel the weight of your heels. Some people may have small narrow feet, but they feel extremely heavy, indicating that the weight of the world bears down on them and to move their feet forward becomes a *drag.* Depression may be an issue. When held, some feet may feel light. This indicates that they may be more enlightened and unburdened or they could also be seeking to escape the physical/emotional issues in their lives and live in the intellectual realm.

We can see how the heels form the basis of our ability to survive and develop into balanced, well-grounded individuals. Any physically painful issues in this area indicate difficulties we may be be having in relation to this.

Chakra Two

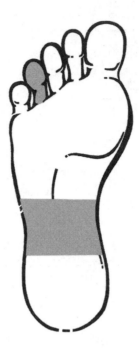

Fig. 13
Second Chakra

"There is no calamity greater than lavish desires.
There is no greater guilt than discontentment.
And there is no greater disaster than greed." Lao Tzu. [1]

Location of actual chakra	Lower abdomen
Location on foot	Just above the heel/lower half of instep and second toe(for toe numbering see next section on toes)
Emotional expression	Guilt
Relationships	To individuals (partners, spouses, children etc.)
Lessons in	Sexuality, abuse, rejection, pleasure or no pleasure, boundaries, money/wealth
Colour	Orange
Related body parts	Bladder, sex organs, lower back, spleen, intestines
Key words	Feeling, need/greed, digesting issues and experiencing
Element	Water

The intestines are located in the second chakra, hence this chakra's relation to elimination. The intestines symbolise our ability to release issues, If we cannot do so, we become emotionally constipated. Constipation comes from the Latin word *constipare*, meaning to cram. If our emotions back up on us, we feel crammed with unresolved feelings.

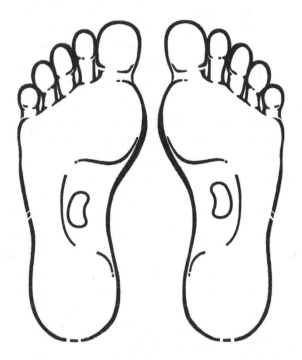

Fig. 14 · Location of the kidneys. (Note: the kidneyarea on the left foot is slightly more raised than on the right foot. Although it falls into the area of the third chakra, it still relates to the second chakra.)

This chakra is also where the kidneys are located. (*see Fig. 14*) Kidneys - release unwanted toxins via urine/water. Water has always been symbolic of emotions, so a swollen kidney area indicates feelings that need to be flushed from our systems. We talk about being *flushed with emotion* indicating that we are full of issues, (probably guilt), that we have been unable to let release. A sunken kidney area indicates that we feel drained and exhausted by the unresolved emotional issues we have not released.

The issues (and not the kidneys) are *draining* us. If this area of your foot is swollen or depressed, ask yourself what feelings you are holding onto?

This section of the foot, together with the upper instep or third chakra, also contains part of the arch of the foot, which symbolises our support issues (also see A–Z section). This is where issues to do with finance arise. Do you feel financially unsupported? Does your backache reflect this? Do you feel supported in your relationships? Steep horizontal ridges in this area of the foot indicate difficulties you may have had to overcome. Very pronounced outer ridges have to do with rigidity and the need for control. Are your boundaries too rigid or not established at all? Are you controlling? Do you manipulate others? How easily do you embrace change? Do you hold determinedly onto the past?

One client had had a series of very difficult relationships, which showed up in the deep lines or ridges across her feet on the lower instep. The resulting lack of self-esteem, together with fear, had caused her to become very controlling, as a way of protecting herself.

As this chakra also concerns both sex and money, it's not hard to see that it's an area that can cause us much pleasure, but also much pain. Both can be used to gain power over another. If there are problems on the lower instep or fourth toe, there may be a sexual dysfunction. Are you sexually cold or do you seek out sexual gratification in order to manipulate others? Pleasure issues and matters of money also are reflected here. Do you deny yourself pleasure to appease your guilt, or are you a hedonistic pleasure-seeking junkie?

One must also remember the interconnectedness of all the chakras as they are, after all, part of the same foot. If the first chakra has problems, it will undoubtedly affect the following chakra, just as having a cut will make walking on the whole foot painful. So we can see that feeling ungrounded (first chakra) may well affect our finances (second chakra). This in turn will affect our self-esteem which is located in the upper instep or third chakra.

Chakra Three

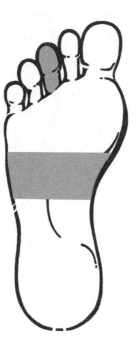

Fig. 15
Third Chakra

*"They must often change who would
be constant in happiness or wisdom."* **Confucius.**[2]

Location of actual chakra	Solar plexus
Location on foot	Upper half of instep, below the ball of the foot and third toe.
Emotional expression	Shame, anger over self-esteem /authoritarian/victim issues. Repressed anger.
Relationships	To self
Lessons in	Self-esteem/self-confidence, responsibility, personal honour, self-discipline, personal power, competition, active/passive behaviour, risk.
Colour	Yellow
Related body parts	Stomach, liver, spleen, pancreas, gall bladder.
Key words	Self, energy, transformation, power, ambition.
Element	Fire

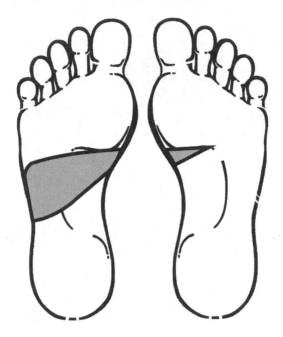

Fig. 16 · Location of the liver

The liver, located mostly on the right (male) side of this area, (*see Fig.16*) was much prized by many primal peoples, who took delight in eating it raw after a kill. The word 'live' is only a letter away from 'liver,' hence this chakra's connection to the amount of life (live) force we have.

The difference between the anger of the first chakra and the third chakra, is that the first chakra or heel's anger involves our physical security, while in the third chakra, our anger is more about our self-esteem being under attack. For instance, if I threaten your safety by brandishing a club, you will switch to fight (anger) or flight (fear) mode. This then is the first chakra in action. If I however, as your colleague, belittle you in the middle of an important presentation to the Board of Directors, the anger you will experience will come from the third chakra. This is where we lash out in *fiery* anger, at our threatened self-esteem. However, anger can be a healthy way of *firing* us up to change. For fire is the element of the third chakra, the transformative energy from where the symbolic Phoenix rises.

Here is where we get *fired up* by a new project, *burn* ourselves *out,* or *burn the candle at both ends*. Where we are bursting with energy or feel very depleted. Alternatively, we may passively accept abuse, while *boiling* internally. We may develop gallstones over situations that *gall* us but do little to express how we really feel. Often our rashness causes us to *burn our fingers*. We have *fire in our bellies*, when we have the energy and enthusiasm to succeed, so that we can *set the world on fire*, or we may have no ambition at all.

The spleen, also found in this part also symbolically expresses anger as in *"venting one's spleen."* The gall bladder here refers to when we don't express our anger, instead we sit with the situation that we find *galling*.

A client of mine has a very fiery personality, with flowing red hair to match her temperament. She is constantly on the go, rushing from one exciting project to the next. Her partner, however, is a very watery personality, who battles to motivate himself to perform even the most mundane of tasks. Such is his emotional problem, that his physical body retains fluid and swells with painful, unexpressed emotions. Here then are the two elements of fire and water that have sought, through this relationship, to reach balance. In reality we need to balance our own water and fire (activity and passivity), to reach our own inner harmonious state. If this chakra is not in balance, the see-saw will tilt either to excessive A-type personality action, or will stagnate and be extremely low-reacting.

In this chakra we can swing between a lack of energy or an excess of it. We can have a *fiery temper* or show little emotion. We may *battle to stomach* situations, resulting in stomach disorders such as acidity and reflux problems. We may be over-disciplined and insist that our way is the right way, or we may lack self-discipline and battle to complete tasks. Our bellies may expand as we attempt to push ourselves out into the world, or we may have collapsed midriffs as we shrink into ourselves.

In practically every religion or belief system, the element of fire is used as part of the ceremonial process. From candles and incense to smudging, fire is seen as purifying and transformative. Fire has transformative energy, consequently from this chakra we can transform ourselves (often through being angry which forces us to act.) We then enter a new stage of being where we live from the heart with unconditional love, both of ourselves and others and leave behind a life lived solely *below the belt*.

Chakra Four

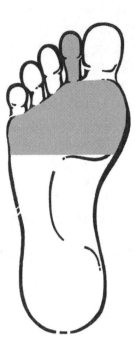

Fig. 17
Fourth Chakra

Location of actual chakra	Heart
Location on foot	The ball of the foot and fourth toe
Emotional expression	Love/grief
Relationships	To others whom we love unconditionally
Lessons in	Self-esteem/self-confidence, responsibility, personal honour, self-discipline, personal power, competition, active/passive behaviour, risk.
Colour	Green
Related body parts	Heart, lungs, breasts, thymus gland, arms, shoulders
Key words	Intimacy, self-acceptance, forgiveness, giving and receiving, critical, lonely, cold, balanced, insensitive, rejection, divorce, head/heart split, relationship fear and unresolved grief
Element	Air

The word 'ball' comes from the Latin word *follis* which refers to something that is blown up or inflated. When our hearts are full of unresolved issues we *puff up our chests*, and in doing so we appear to be *full of ourselves*. We might come across as arrogant or narcissistic, whereas in truth we are covering up for a deep fear of being rejected, or lacking in self-esteem. A swollen ball of the foot, like a puffed up chest, indicates huge unexpressed emotions.

Alternatively, we might deflate ourselves, by being round-shouldered and sunken-chested, as we seek to protect ourselves from criticism and hurt. Are we afraid to reach out and receive love, or do we have problems giving love to those around us? Are we holding onto issues from the past instead of forgiving those involved, (including ourselves) and letting the issue go? Do we feel divided about the roles we live in our lives?

The ball of the foot often looks swollen with unexpressed emotion, or flat and sunken with feelings that drain us. It is not uncommon for the heart to have a vertical dividing line, (*heartbreak*) under the fourth toe, across the ball of the foot, indicating some kind of separation, either as a result of a divorce, being sent away from home or else living a divided life, that may be causing us heartache. Over the actual heart itself, (*see Fig. 18*), or the entire ball of the foot, there is often a hardened piece of skin, or a callus, indicating that life's events have caused us to create a protective barrier around our heart, as in this example:

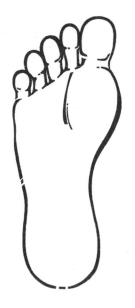

Fig. 18
Heart Chakra with
line dividing it

When examining Lena, the main thing that attracted my attention were the yellow calluses on the heart reflexes, as well as on the heart/lung area of both feet. (*see Fig. 19*)

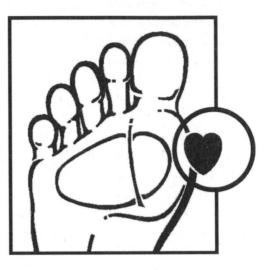

Fig. 19
Calluses on heart and heart reflex. (While the fourth chakra speaks generally of heartfelt issues, the heart reflex is very specific to the actual heart.)

There was a big callus build-up under the second toe on the right foot. Consequently, I felt drawn to ask her if she had been through a divorce, or perhaps experienced some major heartfelt issue that may be the reason for this 'wall.' She said she had recently gone through a divorce. Noticing the yellowness *(see colours of the feet on page 62)* of the larger callus on the right side, I asked her if she was still 'really fed up with her ex-husband. She agreed she was although knew that she should forgive him but, as we all know, it is hard to consciously shift from feeling victimized into accessing the role of victor, as this entails forgiving; and in Caroline Myss's words, *"Forgiveness is not attractive until you get to the other side!"* [3]

I have seen cuts over this heart area to indicate just how *cut-up* a client was about a situation. If it's on the left foot, remember it is affecting the present, or involves females, or the female sides of ourselves; a cut on the right foot would represent the past and relates to men, or the male aspects of ourselves.

One man I recall had large calluses across both the balls of his feet. He confessed that he battled to open up emotionally to his present girlfriend (or indeed with any past girlfriend). In fact, in spite of having many girlfriends, he had never been able to tell anyone he had been with that he loved them, even if he had felt strongly about them. This inability to make himself vulnerable was causing problems in his current relationship.

I asked him if perhaps he feared rejection should he make himself more vulnerable by opening up to her about how he felt. He agreed. We then explored the idea that in order to work through his fear he would have to embrace its opposite – faith. (In other words he would have to start trusting both himself and others.) He admitted having a huge fear of being vulnerable and that fear held him back from being truly open and intimate.

Past childhood experiences also revealed that he had never experienced actual love, instead his environment had been cold and filled with constant criticism when he failed to measure up to his parents' expectations – in particular his strict, often abusive, father. It was not surprising then to discover that he really was not certain what love actually was and how it felt. At this point he became very emotional and sobbed, grieving for the lack of unconditional love in his life. We spoke of the feelings of rejection he experienced when he felt abandoned by his family and sent away to boarding school; he also talked of his violent, bullying, school environment. Other issues emerged where he admitted to shutting down emotionally, rather than experiencing traumatic emotions. As he unburdened himself his feet became lighter and the yellow colouring transformed to a healthier pink. The next and last time I saw him, he told me he had told his girlfriend he loved her and I noticed that some of the calluses had started to peel away. I hope, and trust, the process continued.

When I found myself living a double life, as an advertising manager/designer on the one hand and a Reiki practitioner/artist on the other, a line developed down the ball of my foot, indicating the divide I felt between the life I was living versus the new life I wanted to embrace. Although not an overnight process, as I let go of the one life and embraced the new life, the division lessened. This move made me feel better about who I was and so I was then able to love not only myself more, but all aspects of my life and the people who were a part of it.

This is also where we often find *bruises*, which are deep hurts that have knocked us black and blue, as their colouring indicates. These bruises may make it physically and emotionally painful to move ahead in life.

The first three toes of one woman, who was an alcoholic in recovery, were very small and bent under, compared to her large fourth or heart toe. (*see Fig. 20*)

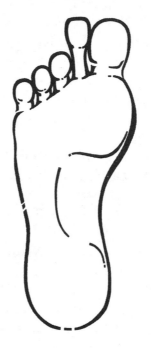

Fig. 20
Funnel shaped fourth
chakra toe

Her addiction had both restricted and lessened her sense of self, so that she had hidden much of who she was from others. Having overcome her addiction, she found herself to be a gifted intuitive and used this ability to assist others in their development. Her funnel-shaped fourth toe (in the area of the seventh chakra on the heart toe) showed how she had developed her ability to channel information.

Having reached the heart and how we experience love, we move on to how we express both love and ourselves, in the fifth chakra.

Chakra Five

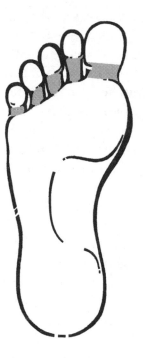

Fig. 21
Fifth Chakra

"Give every man thine ear, but few thy voice;
take each man's censure but reserve thy judgment." **William Shakespeare**.[4]

"In the beginning was the Word, and the Word was with God,
and the word was God. St John ch.1:1.[5]

Location of actual chakra	Throat
Location on foot	Necks of the toes and big toe
Emotional expression	Self-expression, truth/lies
Relationships	Compassion for all
Lessons in	Communication, creativity and truth
Colour	Turquoise
Related body parts	Throat, thyroid, neck, mouth, jaw, ears, teeth and gums
Key words	Listening, whining voice, resonant voice, domineering voice, creative, expressive, toxic speech or gossip, garrulous, speaking one's truth
Element	Ether

Have you ever wanted to speak and found your throat just closed up? Have you got a tickle or developed a cough just as you stood up to make a speech? I once watched a lay minister perform a funeral service before a large audience. Unfamiliar with the congregation and the number of people, he coughed throughout the proceedings, only to speak quite clearly later when the pressure was off. Do you sit mutely afraid to express your views? Do you find yourself lying, either to yourself, or to others, about issues? Do you long to express your creative potential, but are afraid to do so? Are you shy and retiring, or are you garrulous and never let anyone else get a word in edgeways? Did you, as a child, have someone else's perception of their truth *rammed down your throat?* Do you *voice your feelings?*

This is the centre from where we speak things into being, where we can transmute the baseness of the lower chakras into the gold of the divine. It is from this centre that we can assume the role of magician or alchemist and create our own reality (provided it does not interfere with our karma). We may have assumed the role of an artist in the third chakra in order to work with our feelings, but in the fifth chakra we are what we create. In other words, we become not only the creator but the masterpiece as well.

"We are the canvas and as such, are both the creator and the creation." [6]

The longer the toe necks are, the greater a person's artistic/creative *potential is*, indicating they have greater ability to draw in concepts and ideas. This does not mean that someone with short toes has no artistic abilities, but rather their ability will perhaps lie more in realism, than conceptualism.

When the toes are bent under (often giving the appearance that they are gripping Mother Earth,) it is an indication of the creative potential we have, but are not using. Creativity in this context does not refer simply to art, but to all areas where we create something from nothing, be it a company, a gourmet meal, a garden or recreating ourselves. The reasons we hide our creative potential are numerous. These could include the fear of stepping into our power (getting to *grips* with the project, as the curled toes mirror getting a grip on the earth), or from the fear of failing, holding ourselves back from achieving because we don't want to appear to rise above others, or because we lack confidence in ourselves and consequently belittle our ideas.

Bent toes might also show that we cannot *stand up* for our ideas and beliefs, as in the client below:

The toes on her left foot were scrunched up, while on the right foot, the toes were straighter, indicating that whatever the problem was it was either worse in the present or more to do with female energy. I mentioned to her the broad scenarios above and asked her if she ever felt as if those around her suppressed ideas. She immediately identified with this concept, especially in relation to her mother who was scornful of her daughter's new holistic, spiritual approach to life. My client said that she had always *bowed down* to her mother's beliefs and never voiced her own.

Seeing the necks of the toes constricted, particularly on the left side, I followed up this statement further by asking if she felt it difficult to express her feelings to her mother. She admitted she did, although she occasionally did loose her temper and say things she regretted. She was also unable to express her feelings about religion and spirituality. Now she was afraid to voice these feelings because she did not want to hurt or upset the old woman, fearing that there might be health implications if she did. We spoke at length about how this pattern was blocking, not just her expression to her mother, but her ability to express herself in general. In time, I hoped that she would be able to understand that her mother merely mirrored all the ideas and concepts that she felt afraid to make manifest.

Creativity is not only about art, it can manifest in many forms, as I discovered in the case of a young man in his early thirties, who came to see me. A short, slightly tubby guy very casually dressed and in his early thirties, his appearance did not convey the wealth that he had already ammassed. I noticed he had extremely long toe necks and asked if he was very creative or artistic. He disagreed with this, yet the toe necks implied a man who was filled with conceptual and creative ability. I was confused and passed onto other aspects of his feet to see where that would lead. We spoke about his career and life in general. He was clearly highly skilled at creating money, with his various entrepreneurial schemes. At the age of thirty he had achieved what few people ever manage, in that he did not *have* to work. It then occurred to me that he was literally the alchemist or magician (the archetype of the fifth chakra). He could turn base metal into gold. (Literally, unused land and bricks into palatial homes and gold for himself.) Making money was his way of being extremely creative. He agreed with this concept and said it explained the relative ease he had had accumulating wealth. The acknowledgement of his ability gave him a greater sense of self-worth.

Now that you have some understanding of the symbology of the toe necks, you can look at which specific chakra the aspect of the foot you are interested in, falls. Linking the two aspects will give you a clearer picture of what is going on. Look at the undersides of your toe necks. Are they constricted, as in the case of the woman in the example above? Do they have deep lines? This could mean that we feel strangled by ourselves and others when it comes to expressing ourselves. It's as if the idea gets stuck, like a lump in our throat. Alternatively, we say what we feel other people want us to say and do not express our own truth.

Once we have mastered the power to create and manifest our ideas, we are ready to go within and establish the answer to the question, "Who am I?"

Chakra Six

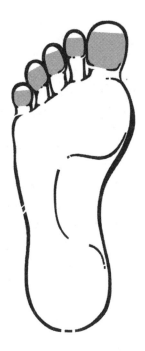

Fig. 22
Sixth Chakra

Location of actual chakra	Between the eyebrows on the forehead
Location on foot	Lower parts of toe pads
Emotional expression	Insight/intuition/illusion
Relationships	To inner self

38

Lessons in	Recognizing our own patterns or not being aware of them. Denial/delusion/ trusting intuition
Colour	Indigo blue
Related body parts	Pituitary gland, eyes, ears
Key words	Perception, wisdom, inner vision, under- standing, sensitivity or insensitivity to the subtle, visualization, imagination, obsessive behaviour, memory functions, seeing events from a symbolic perspec- tive, channelling, psychic abilities, medi- tation, and concentration.
Element	Light

There is a quote, along the lines of "if you don't go within, you will go without." Never were there truer words, for if we don't reflect or become aware of our patterns, we will continue to repeat them endlessly. Going around and around in circles does not allow us to make much progress in life (this incarnation) which is why understanding ourselves is so important if we are to evolve. We do this through accessing our dreams, quiet meditation or contemplation, using our intuitive abilities to access what is going on and symbolically seeing what is happening. From this, we gain the wisdom that will eventually help us to move beyond the cycle of our karma and into the seventh chakra.

A friend mentioned the other day how emotionally hard it was see- ing and owning her patterns, to the point that she was actively avoid- ing doing so. It's easy to understand why most of us settle for this option. However, the price to pay is the conscious awareness that we are inviting the old ways of being into our lives, instead of moving ahead. The work is hard and takes courage and, at times, the rewards seem insignificant compared to the emotional effort; but the reward eventually does appear, often when you least expect it, or just when you are ready to throw in the towel.

The size of the pads is significant in that the larger the toe pad, the greater *potential* there may be for thoughts, intellectual activity, ideas and concepts. This does not mean that someone with small pads will not have such potential, just that it may come *easier* to someone with bigger pads. However, in the end, it's what we make of what we have been given and how we move ahead.

Often *sinusitis* sufferers will have toe pads where the base is more pointed (*see Fig. 23*) indicating that we ourselves, or those around us, are blocking our creative concepts, thoughts and ideas, just as our physical sinuses are blocked. This causes us to feel irritated with ourselves or with others, as our inflamed sinuses demonstrate. Excessive watery fluids in the body are also a sign of emotions that we are holding onto, so there may be much pain and sadness in being unable to truly see and release where we have become stuck.

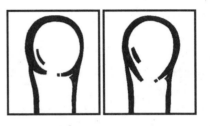

Fig. 23
The toe on the left is normal; the one on the right has a teardrop appearance at the base of the pad and can often be an indication of sinus.

Through gaining insight into ourselves, we are ready to clear out the old and make way for a new way of being. We are ready for the seventh chakra, where our connection to the divine inspiration of our thoughts allows us to move through life fully conscious.

Chakra Seven

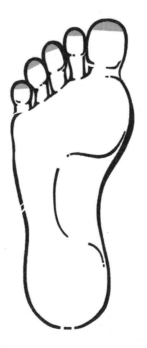

Fig. 24
Seventh Chakra

40

"I decided that it was not wisdom that enabled [poets] to write their poetry, but a kind of instinct or inspiration, such as you find in seers and prophets who deliver all their sublime messages without knowing in the least what they mean." Socrates. [7]

Location of actual chakra	Top of head
Location on foot	Tips of toe pads
Emotional expression	Wisdom and attachment
Relationships	To God/the Divine, Allah, Jehovah, etc.
Lessons in	Living in the moment, grace, non-attachment and selflessness
Colour	Violet/white
Related body parts	Hair, central nervous system, brain
Key words	Let go and let God. Universal understanding, spiritual intelligence, transcendence, mastery, ability to analyze, open to new ideas, wisdom, divine union or *union mystico*, over-intellectualization, fanaticism, learning difficulties, cynicism and guru.
Element	All thoughts

What we have more than any other creature, plant or mineral is free will. The more we reconnect with God or the Divine, the more we relinquish free will to make true the phrase from the Lord's prayer "thy will be done," (as opposed to my will.) The seventh chakra is where we open ourselves up to receiving Divine guidance and thoughts. Some fortunate people actually have pads that are shaped liked funnels, indicating how open they are to receiving from the universe. (The good news is that our feet constantly change and so we all have potential to become greater receptors, if we use the thoughts and ideas that are given to us, just as a muscle grows in strength the more we exercise it.)

The various sections or chakras, can be seen to be a kind of Jacob's Ladder, up which we can ascend to become whole. We need, in the seventh chakra, to learn to break free from attachments to ideas, beliefs and things (be they people or objects) for it is our attachments that bind us. When we have mastered this chakra we would not only have knowledge of ourselves but also all that is. Consequently, we can choose to transcend the physical plane. Few of us however reach this level of adepthood. Therefore, we are left to deal with the more mundane aspects of this chakra, such as having our thoughts invalidated, being forced into belief systems we know don't relate to us and fearing to question what we are told.

We may have calluses over the tops of our toes as we try to protect ourselves from those who may belittle our ideas. Our toe pads might appear swollen if our heads burst with all the ideas we have not yet manifested. If the toe pads are squashed or bunched up we may have no time or space where we can think for ourselves.

In order for anything to be created, an idea has to be conceived. To understand how this idea becomes manifest (or where it gets blocked) we need to understand its passage through the chakras. Here is a rough model of how it works:

If we receive an idea/guidance via the tip of the big toe (seventh chakra) we may gain insight into it via the pads (sixth chakra) and then we could start to express it via the toe necks (fifth chakra). On the second toe (fourth chakra) we would need to ask whether our heart was in the concept, while on the third toe (third chakra) we would ask ourselves what impact the success or failure would have on us and what action we needed to take to make it a reality. On the fourth toe (second chakra) we would look at the financial/relationship implications; and finally we would give the idea roots in our society (see small toe, first chakra.)

Consequently, each chakra has its role to play, as we channel through ideas and thoughts from the Divine or Mental realm and manifest them onto this physical plane.

A note on the numbering of the toes

The way we number the toes when we refer to them in the book is opposite to conventional numbering. (Even though it's traditional to refer to the big toe as the first toe and so on, for the purposes of keeping each toe corresponding to the chakra it represents, we will reverse the process.)

As can be seen in the diagrams for the seven chakras above, the first five chakras also include a toe. This is because each toe represents not only the fifth, sixth and seventh chakras, namely the neck of the toes, the toe pads and the top of pads but also relates to one of the other five chakras.

Common toe numbering

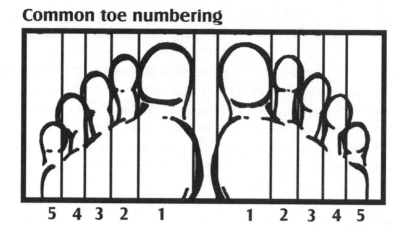

Fig. 25 · Chart to show the opposite numbering of the chakras on the toes to common numbering (normally the big toe is called the first toe and so on.)

Chakra numbering vertically and horizontally

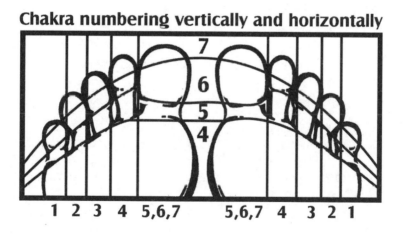

Fig. 26 · How the toes relate to the head

So the little toe, for instance, relates not only to the fifth, sixth and seventh chakras but also to the first *(see Fig. 25)*. Whereas the second toe in the diagram, corresponds to the second chakra in relation to the fifth, sixth and seventh chakras.

In order to explain this further, imagine that the toe pads all represent small heads, with each head representing a different aspect of the sixth and seventh chakra, depending on the toe involved, yet still carrying the overall concept or symbol of what the head represents *(see Fig. 26)*.

Once you relate to this next bit of visual imagery, you will be further along the path to understanding this chakra. The big toe on the left foot makes up only half a face, but together with the right toe, the 'head' is complete, giving us nine 'heads' in all.

If the toes in general can be seen to represent where we express, gain insight and ideas/concepts respectively, then each specific toe will relate to where we express, gain insight and ideas/concepts respectively in relation to what the chakra concerned represents. For instance, the second toe relates to the fourth chakra, consequently we can see that expression, insight and ideas/concepts respectively are relevant to and are about love, intimacy, self-love and integration. It is similar to checking co-ordinates on a bar chart.

In the following chapter we will take a look at how to examine your own feet.

CHAPTER 3

Solemates

Becoming buddies with your feet

How do you feel about your feet?

It might sound like a strange question, but many of us have very firm ideas about our feet. Some of my clients hate their feet to the point of refusing to be seen barefoot, while others adore their feet and spend loads of money having them pampered and petted. Let's do a very quick and simple exercise that lets you become aware of your relationship to your feet:

PART TWO: (Don't read part two until you've completed part one.) Find a paper and pen and just sit still for a moment to give yourself time to reflect on the question "How do I feel about my feet?" Then write down your thoughts, no matter how absurd they may seem to be. Maybe there are aspects that appeal and certain ones that don't? Perhaps you used to like your feet, but have since changed your mind? Don't rush the process; just write down all the thoughts about your feet. Start with "my feet are..." and then write whatever pops into your mind. Here are some examples:

My feet are... so big and clumsy, and my toes aren't straight. I definitely prefer keeping them covered! I hate my feet. I always have. I keep them hidden. My bent second toe is the worst part and I also dislike how my toe nails have become so thick. They are also very big and I seem to feel they will trip me up the whole time. Perhaps that is why I am so clumsy.

My feet are... great. I am comfortable with them. I feel they are attractive, sort of long and elegant. They are a part of my body that makes me feel really good. They haven't aged or wrinkled like the rest of me has. My toes are really long and I like that.

PART ONE: When you feel you have completed the exercise and have written all you can about your feet, you're ready to go to the next stage of the exercise. Now replace the words "my feet are..." with "I am ..." So the first example would read:

Example I

I am... so big and clumsy, and my toes aren't straight. I definitely prefer keeping them covered, etc.

Some of the insights will be straightforward, but some may need a little more knowledge of what aspects the different parts of the feet relate to; so you will need to refer back to Chapter Two to find out more. Here are the insights derived from the two examples above, with the feedback from both clients.

I am so... big and clumsy
    ("Yes I guess I do feel that about myself.").

... and my toes aren't straight. (Toe necks represent self-expression.)
    ("Being so bent I can see that I battle to express myself and my creativity.").

I definitely prefer keeping them covered
    ("I hide my true self.").

I hate my feet. I always have. I keep them hidden.
    ("I hate myself - probably for not being able to express who I am. I never feel good enough and shut myself off from relationships.").

The bent fourth toe is the worst part. (The fourth toe has to do with the expression of the heart and love/grief).
    ("I struggle to love myself and therefore find intimacy with others a problem as I can't express love to myself or anyone else. This makes me hurt really

badly sometimes. I am afraid of failure and rejection in a relationship and I can't seem to stand up for myself and just get down-trodden").

... and I also dislike how my toe nails have become so thick. (Toe nails are our protection. When thickened they indicate that we have put on a thick layer to shut the world away and protect ourselves).

("I dislike the wall I have built around myself that protects me from feeling vulnerable because I can't get really close to anyone.").

They are also very big and I seem to feel they will trip me up the whole time. Perhaps that is why I am so clumsy. (Big feet, in proportion to the body, can make a big impression in the world. However, with big feet we may also be prone to "put our feet in it.").

("I do feel this is the case with me. I always seem to be saying the wrong thing at the wrong time, which makes me feel even worse about myself and want to retreat more into my thickened nail shell.").

Through this dialogue with her feet, the above person was able to see where her major issues lay. By working with these issues on an emotional and physical level, such as having a pedicure or foot reflexology, she was able to start the process of liking her feet and enjoying the intimacy of having another person massage them. In time she started to feel more comfortable with other people seeing her feet and started to open herself up to the world emotionally as well as beginning to express what she felt. It was a long process, but in time her toes began to uncurl and she actually became proud of herself and the impression she was able to make in the world.

Example 2

My feet are... great. I am comfortable with them. I feel they are attractive, sort of long and elegant. They are a part of my body that makes me feel really good. They haven't aged like the rest of my skin has. My toes are really long and I like that.

I am... great. I am comfortable with them.
    (*myself – who I am*).

(*I am*) attractive, long and elegant.
 (*either tall in actual height, or in mental standing*).

(*I*)... feel good
 (*about myself*).

(*I*) haven't aged like the rest of my skin has.
 (*Skin is what we show to the outside world or how the outside world sees us. Perhaps I feel young inside*).

My toes are really long and I like that.
 (*Long toes show creative ability and ability to express one's ideas and concepts and the ability to stand tall/stand-up for one's beliefs*).

This person's view of herself was clearly very different; with the fourth toe longer than the big toe, she would have leadership abilities; she would, however, need to be wary of wanting to dominate and become self-opinionated. In this case the person concerned had done much work on herself in terms of releasing her emotional baggage, and genuinely felt at peace with who she was, as opposed to having an inflated opinion born out of feelings of inadequacy. This foot reading affirmed to her the positive aspects of the work she had done, and by her own admission, she may have felt differently about her feet in the past.

This is a simple way of getting to understand how you feel about yourself. If your comments were similar to the first example, you would now have a clue as to where your feelings of self-dislike might be coming from. You might be angry or ashamed with yourself for not expressing your true feelings and thoughts, both to yourself and to others. You may be resentful with those people who you might feel have held you back or forced you into their way of thinking. Understanding this now allows you to work on this issue, so that you can arrive at the point when you can fully embrace all aspects of yourself lovingly.

To do this you may need to turn around the description of your feet to their opposite meaning to affirm the positive changes that this understanding will make in your life. Thus: "I prefer being *open* with my thoughts," instead of "I prefer keeping them *covered*." "I hate my feet/self" would become "I love myself." "My toe necks (expression) are not straight" would become "My way of expressing myself is clear and straight-forward." "I am big and clumsy (unconscious)" might be turned around to "I am powerful; I stand tall and act consciously." Be gentle with yourself. Some of these issues may have walked with you for years; realize that the time has now come to change that way of being. Your feet are the messengers from your soul. Don't shoot the messenger!

Life and soul

In searching your feet to find some answers to yourself and your life, remember that there are no such things as "good or bad" feet. There are simply conditions and experiences that have caused you to respond in a certain way. Looking back over our lives, we have all responded and behaved in a myriad of different ways. The advantage of being conscious of the why's and the wherefore's empowers us to make the choice of moving beyond the need to act in a certain way. For instance, if we can recognize via our very high arched foot that we have a need for perfection (and consequently lose excessive energy attempting to be perfect) our awareness, or confirmation and acceptance of what we are, allows us to change.

Write down a dialogue with your feet under the headings:

Aspect examined (such as corn, cut, wrinkle, etc)

> **The issue**
> **My need is**
> **The outcome of this need**
> **The truth is**
> **The result is**

Aspect examined: High-arched foot/perfectionism: We can start a dialogue with ourselves like this:

> **The issue:** Okay, I acknowledge I have a need for perfection.
> **My need is:** I also want others to be perfect and it causes me frustration when they aren't.
> **The outcome of this need:** If everyone were perfect then life would be great.
> **The truth is:** They and I are not perfect (by my standards at least).
> **The result:** Therefore, while I remain needing everyone and

everything, myself included, to be perfect, I live in frustration. That does not serve me and wastes energy.

My new truth: I will therefore stop expecting everyone to be perfect and accept him/her, and myself, as we are. Each time I find this old need reappearing, I will remind myself of this.

Here is another example:

Aspect examined: Bent toes/difficulty in expressing what you believe or who you are: A dialogue might go like this:

> **The issue:** I have a problem when it comes to expressing myself.
> **My need is:** To have the courage to say what I feel.
> **The outcome of this need:** I would not feel ashamed and angry with myself.
> **The truth is:** I am afraid to do so.
> **The result:** I withdraw and bend to other's beliefs. My toes mirror this.
> **My new truth:** I say what I mean and speak my truth. Doing so means I no longer need to feel ashamed. Because I say what I mean, I love myself more and so do others.

Using statements like these will give you the opportunity of coming to new truths about yourself and letting go of old and past beliefs about yourself.

How to examine your own feet

It's easy to look at the tops of your feet, but harder to see the soles, so using a mirror is helpful. A digital camera can also be useful, but it can't record the subtle changes in the feet as you work with each chakra. However, for placement of warts, calluses etc. a camera is a simple way to keep a record of how your feet alter over time as you work with issues.

Another option is to sit with your knees pointed outwards and your feet turned inwards. You should be able to see most of your soles this way. The only problem with this is that the twisted feet often show ridges etc. that would not normally be there, but it's a great way to look more closely at corns, calluses, and cuts.

Note: throughout the book the toes are reffered to by the traditional numbering and not the chakra numbering. E.g. the fourth toe describes the second chakra and the big or first toe chakras five, six and seven.

Otherwise having a friend draw your feet and record any markings for you to investigate later, is another way to examine your feet.

REMEMBER, the feet are very revealing, so be gentle with yourself and with all the bumps and lumps you may find. They are part of what has made your life's journey so unique. Even if they are painful, bent, twisted or callused, the feet are simply reminding you that it may not have been an easy path that you've already walked, and in this you are not alone.

Allow yourself time and space to acknowledge that. Then, when you are ready, make the decision to move on and shed what no longer nurtures you.

CHAPTER 4

Soul Searching

General observations of the feet
Foot shapes and what they mean

The difference between the left foot and the right foot

We talk freely about left-brained and right-brained people and the significance of being one or the other. The feet are also significant in terms of left and right, although the attributes between the left and right hemispheres of the brain, are opposite on the rest of the body, including the feet. This is because the nerve ganglia crosses over in the head so that, for instance, if someone has a stroke on the left side of their body, they may experience a headache on the right side of their head, and vice versa.

Whereas a right-brained person would be more visual, creative and carry feminine attributes that are stronger - such as intuition - the right side of the body relates to the more masculine attributes such as linguistic and/or analytical skills and also physical strength. The feet follow the body as opposed to the head, so left feet relate to the female aspects of ourselves, as well as to relationships with women and our mothers. Left feet also represent the present and what is going on now in our lives. Shadow aspects of ourselves (the parts that we keep hidden from others) may also show up more clearly on the left foot. The right foot, as with the right side of the body, refers to the male aspects of ourselves as well as interaction with men and our fathers. The right foot is also about the past and events linked to the past.

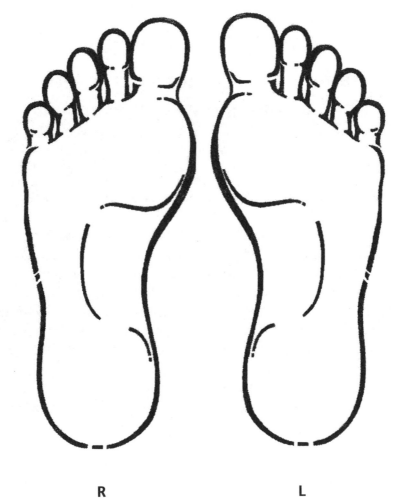

R   L

Fig. 27
Left foot female
Right foot male

Here then are the guides as to which organs are mirrored in what location on the feet.

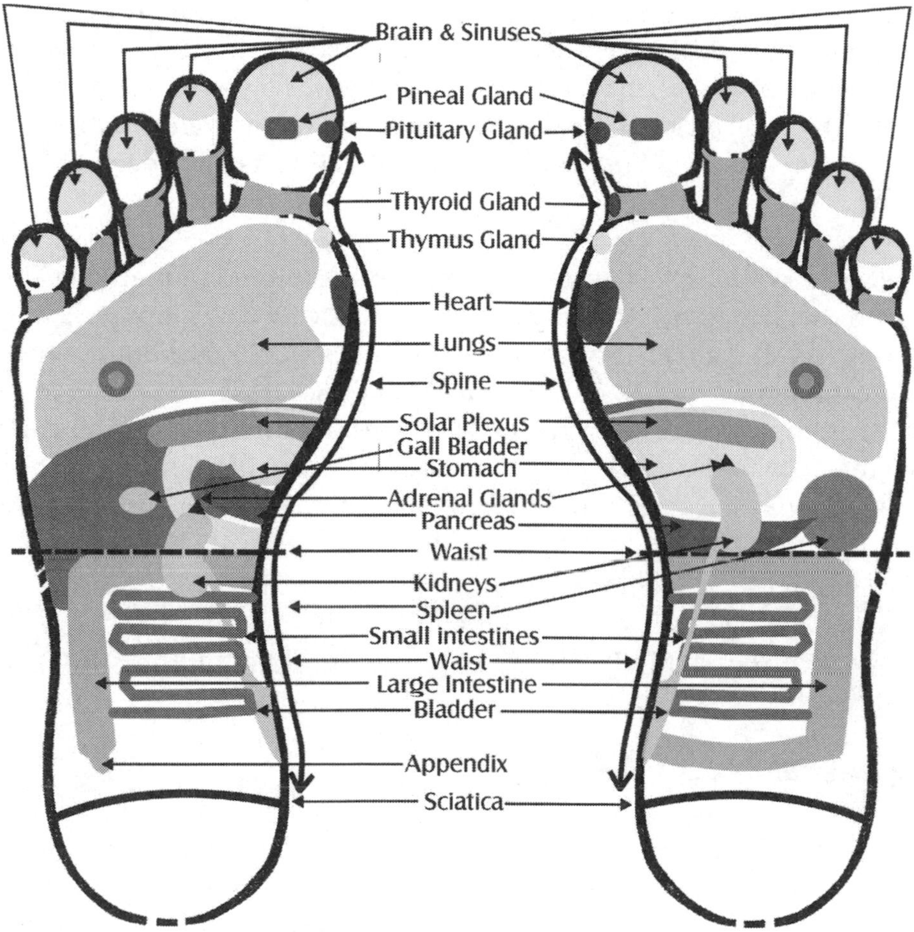

Fig. 28
Illustration depicting the parts of the body
and their location on the feet

As in the body, the organs reflected on the feet fall on the male and female sides, with the exception of the spleen, which is on the left foot only, just as in the body. In medieval physiology, the spleen was considered to be the 'seat of morose feelings and bad temper,' a trait somehow ascribed to the fairer sex. Have you heard the phrase *venting your spleen*? Clearly, this is a way of ridding oneself of these irritations and could well explain its location on the left foot only! Louise Hay in her book *Heal Your Body*[2] links the spleen to obsessions which, while clearly an issue with both sexes, may be found more in the feminine side of us all. A healthy spleen rids the blood of impurities, allowing us each to be more compassionate and sympathetic, as well as being clearer in our being.

The liver, while reflected on both feet, is more predominant on the right foot. The liver has long been associated with raw emotions, warrior energy and anger. (Native American tribes would take out the liver of a captured foe and eat it raw, as a symbol for taking on the life force of their enemy.) The liver gives our bodies life force, hence the close resemblance to the word "live." Men are known to have more fire than women, who have more water. Fire is action and anger - often male principles. It is not surprising then that Chinese medicine relates the liver to anger and repressed anger.

The heart can be seen more predominantly on the left side, which shows how our emotions are related more to the feminine aspects of ourselves.

Big Feet and Small Feet

People with large feet in proportion to their bodies have the potential to create a *big impression* in this life (can also be a reference to the footprint they leave behind and suggests they are very grounded in this life, although they may also be prone to *putting their foot in it)*.

People with proportionally smaller feet, may have a quieter, more reserved approach to life as they *tread lightly* on their path. While they may create an impact on the world around them, it will be gentler and perhaps less forceful and dynamic than their larger-footed pals.

Five types of feet

Feet vary enormously in length, width, overall shape and characteristics. However, as a starting point, I will identify five main categories which, very broadly speaking, gives us an overall view of the personalities of those involved. It must be emphasized that due to variations in toe length, etc., this view is very general.

The Greek or Morton's foot

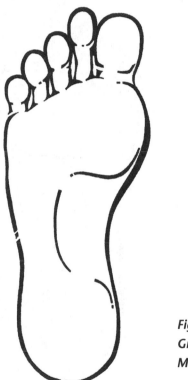

Fig. 29
Greek or
Morton's foot

In this type of foot, the heart (fourth) toe is longer than the big toe, or there may be a deeper space between the two toes. The width of the foot varies from narrow to medium (approximately 20% of the population have this type of foot).

MEANING: This type of foot shows a strong need to lead. Can inspire others to greatness by putting themselves and their ideas out there. More of a thinker than a doer, though can be both.

The Egyptian foot

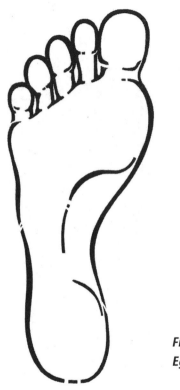

Fig. 30
Egyptian foot

This type of foot has the big toe longer than the second toe. Like the Greek foot, it also ranges in width between narrow and medium.

MEANING: Great ideas and concepts. A visionary, but because the big toe is vulnerable to scuffing, it means that sometimes the ideas which the visionary puts out into the world make him/her vulnerable to criticism. If the heel is small compared to the ball of the foot, as in the example, the person may battle with grounding their ideas and consequently may have financial issues.

The Giselle or Peasant foot

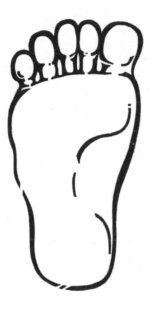

Fig. 31
Giselle or Peasant foot

Here at least three toes are the same length and all of them tend to be short and square. The foot width itself ranges from medium to wide.

MEANING: Solid. Down to earth and reliable. Well-grounded. Salt of the earth! Would rather deal with day-to-day issues than speculating about the future. Hard-working person.

Scottish/Irish foot

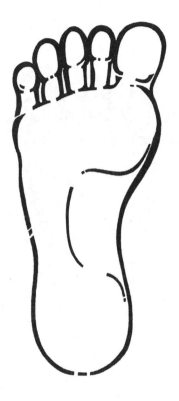

Fig. 32
Scottish or
Irish foot

Much like the Giselle foot, however it is long and narrow with toes that are almost in a straight line at the top, or square.

MEANING: Airy nature. Sensitive and caring. May battle to broaden horizons and as such may be quite conservative. Change is not something they find easy. Consistent in their thoughts and emotions.

**Modern
English
foot**

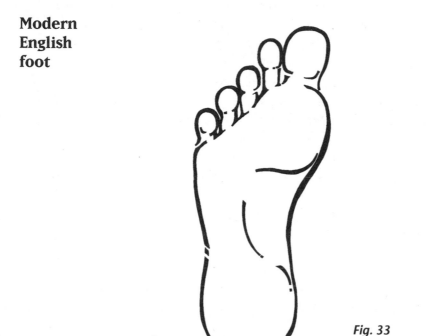

*Fig. 33
Modern English foot*

This foot is wider than the Scottish/Irish type, with the toes sloping down sharply.

MEANING: Stable and down to earth, with not as much emphasis placed on developing the spiritual and creative aspects of self, or a reluctance to express ideas and thoughts relating to these issues. Would rather choose to withdraw than say the wrong thing.

Colours of feet

While we may consider our feet to be the same colour as the rest of our body, they do have subtle variations and this detail gives us more insight into our state of being.

RED AREAS: Indicates where we may be angry. For instance if the red area is on the heel, we know from Chapter Two that this area relates to family, society or work-related issues. So it would likely reflect that it is in relation to these areas where we feel angry. It is not wrong to feel anger. Where it causes us dis-ease is when we bottle it up and don't express it. Throwing violent temper tantrums comes as a result of not expressing our anger and then like a boiling kettle the feelings explode, often over a small incident. This is as harmful as withdrawing into festering disapproval. Simply finding the courage to state calmly why you are angry at the time is an effective way to ensure that you don't bottle things up. "I find what you are doing offensive and here is why," is one way of saying what we feeling. We are often afraid to say how we feel in case we offend others, whereas by not saying how we feel, we offend ourselves.

YELLOW AREAS: Yellow patches, or whole feet which are yellow show us that we are generally fed up with a situation or person, depending on where exactly the yellow is located. If it's over the entire foot it may be that we are fed up with our lives in general. Often found on calluses, yellow there would show we are fed up with creating a barrier around our feelings. When people are allowed to express their frustration, the yellow will often fade.

WHITE AREAS: If your feet are white, it's time to book that holiday! You are exhausted and washed out. Clearly life situations or events are exhausting you. Put your feet up, smell the roses, nurture yourself.

BLUE AREAS: Are you tired from all the pain and hurt in your life? Do you feel hurt or bruised by people or situations in your life? Whenever we feel bruised, we are feeling hurt and in need of comfort. Are you taking time to give to yourself? You do not have to suffer. You can stand up for yourself. If life is hurting you, what can you do to change the situation?

Asymmetrical feet

It is said that we spend much of our lives seeking balance. Feet that dif-fer greatly in size are less likely to have owners who have balanced male and female aspects.

Hormone imbalances, while still in utero, can cause babies to be born who may subsequently grow up with one foot larger than the other.[1] Initially this sounds preposterous. However, if we apply the theory of 'as above so below' perhaps this research is not as outlandish as it may appear. If the feet mirror our bodies and emotions, and if our feet are out of balance (i.e. one bigger than the other) then surely we could rea-sonably say that our male/female aspects could also be out of balance. This could undoubtedly lead us to jealous behaviour. We would not trust the opposite aspect of ourselves and the larger of the two feet in its fear would seek to govern or control the lesser part.

We also know that hormone imbalances in the womb can create children with hands and feet that are not proportional. Unbalanced pre-partum nurturing frequently leads to imbalance of both the physi-cal and emotional bodies.

By examining which foot is larger, one is able to determine what aspect of that person's self, i.e. male or female, is more dominant. As we have learned, the left foot represents the female, both internally and externally, as well as the present, while the right foot represents the male aspects of ourselves, and the past. Now most people will have slightly larger features on the right side (from breasts, to hands, to legs, and to feet) this is not surprising, given that we live in a traditionally male-dominated society. We aspire to goals, achieving and getting out there, as opposed to going within, being accepting, and allowing. As the feet also represent the past and present, a smaller left foot would indicate being restrained or confined either in our feminine nature or in the present, or if the right were to be smaller, then we may have been more restrained in the past or, alternatively, aspects of our male self may be less expressed.

Not being in balance with our own male and female aspects may reflect in our outer relationships.

CHAPTER 5

Relating not Dictating

On your toes

"The unexamined life is not worth living." **Socrates.**[1]

"The meeting of two personalities is like the contact of two chemical substances; if there is any reaction, both are transformed." **Karl Gustav Jung.**[2]

The feet, as you are discovering, are very revealing about a person's psyche. Having examined your own feet and come to an understanding about them, you may wish to look at the feet of your friends, family, or clients. If you are not an experienced holistic practitioner or counselor, do so with caution. It can be very damaging to grab a pal's foot and start waxing lyrical about all their 'faults,' or to imply that their poor thinking has resulted in whatever issue they are having to deal with.

When reading the feet of friends or partners, remember that any act involving realization is a sacred one. Treat it as such, i.e. with *no* judgment, only with love and compassion for the pain or struggle that that person may have endured. Those of you who are holistic practitioners will already be doing this; however, given the insight possible with this tool, if not practiced with integrity and empathy, can do more harm than good.

When looking at someone's feet, create a broad framework and then allow the person, whose foot you are looking at, the dignity to fill in the details themselves. You could say something like, "I notice that you have very deep ridges or folds in the area of relationships. Ridges can mean that we have not had a smooth ride, just as walking across a flat surface is easier than climbing up and down hills. Can you relate to this feeling?" Ask questions and listen to the answers with compassion, allowing the other person to find their own meaning and interpretation. This is not a tool to get even, to say "I told you so," or to enter someone's emotional space as an enthusiastic voyeur.

Put your ego and judgment aside and with it the need to be right. This is also not about how clever you can be seen to be, rather it's to help another human being acknowledge areas where they carry their emotional burdens. Through doing so you allow them to release what they feel is appropriate; You are merely facilitating (as opposed to controlling) *their* process to become lighter, happier and more enlightened. Often just having someone listen to our experiences can go a long way towards us releasing them. Also, if someone is not ready to forgive, let go, or accept an issue, respect their choice. It may not be appropriate for them at the moment.

If you have no training as a counsellor and want to examine people's feet, it make be wise to consider taking a counselling course.

Intuition

While many issues on the feet are clearly visible, I rely on my intuition when it comes to which issues to focus on. The feet often almost "speak" to you and draw you to a particular aspect. I have learnt to go with this and let the feet and the client be my guide. Sometimes an area will show up almost glowing, or else a feature that you may have overlooked initially, begs your attention. I feel that its often worth-while to spend more time working with a particular issue in someone's life, and go really deeply into that, rather than be a sort of fortune teller and highlight many issues, while not really assisting the person to let go and clear any of them.

Many people say that they are not intuitive. I believe we all are intuitive; it's just that we often don't trust our intuitive ability. We would sooner go with what our heads or previous experience with others has taught us, rather than listen to that inner voice that is trying to help us.

Often intuition is illogical and if we are very rational and logical in our thinking, we may discard a brilliant intuitive insight because it does not conform to our logic. Another reason we discard insight about our own lives, is because it often means having to change the way we live, and we all know how much we love change! So, rather than be open to our intuition, our ego blocks that inner prompt so we don't have to change.

Intuition is also reliant on our self-esteem. If we don't feel confident within ourselves, we won't trust either our abilities or ourselves. Therefore, we may receive guidance but not trust it sufficiently to act on it. So often we know what to do, but doing it terrifies us and so we ignore our guidance and revert to logic. The only way to improve our trust in our intuition is to act upon it and, when we are rewarded, our belief in our ability and in our inner knowing is strengthened.

Many people will say that they are unable to distinguish between intuition and nonsense. This can be tricky, but in time you will sense the difference between knowing and guessing. Asking your client questions is a good way of feeling if you have correctly interpreted your intuition.

These days many people believe in the idea that one's thinking causes your illnesses. In as much as the subtle (emotions) affects the gross (the body) this may be so, but karma can also play a role in one's pre-allotment when it comes to illness. Often the insight is repeated, with little or no compassion, making someone feel guilty for the fact that they have a problem and eroding their self-esteem further. Whilst the idea that our minds/emotions/bodies are interlinked is true, there are exceptions and if we jump to conclusions, the person whose feet we are pontificating about, has every right to remove themselves and our knee-caps!

When using your intuition with others, ask a question rather than making a statement, to gain a feeling as to whether your intuition is correct. Their response will confirm or negate your insight. For instance, you may sense the heart area of the foot is feeling burdened and sore. Rather than saying, "Oh boy, you really do have a problem with your love-life," you may ask, "It feels to me as if there are unresolved issues in the heart area, does that resonate with you?" Now you empower the person to relate to your question in any way they feel able to. It's *relating* rather than *dictating*, and it allows the client to come to his or her own insights and understanding and you merely act as a guide. Any other way of relating lends itself to disempowering the other person, making them feel reliant on you for the answers. It is unreasonable, then, to expect them to assume any responsibility for their own healing process.

Remember, sometimes people may not be ready to answer. Your understanding and intuition may be 100% correct, yet they may just not be ready to accept the idea. I have had experiences of people rejecting issues only to have them be expressed and accepted later in a follow-up session. That's fine. Everything happens as and when it needs to. There is no right and wrong time. We have to trust and sometimes that's not easy to do!

I recall seeing the image of the Grim Reaper all the time I worked on a client. I immediately jumped to the conclusion that this must be an indication of her imminent death, so said nothing. Only later, as she was leaving, she revealed that it was the first anniversary of her mother's death. My intuition was trying to tell me that. Had I asked her if there was any significance with death on that day, an opportunity may have arisen where she was able to release some of her grief. Instead, by not asking her, I had attempted to control the session (albeit with the best intention and my rescuer archetype at play) and the opportunity was lost. That time I had to forgive myself.

Most often, a session will run itself if you release control of what is happening and trust the process. The most beneficial sessions are those when the person discovers for themselves the issues behind issues. The "Ah Ha!" outcome is far more profound then, both in the client's experience of it and the healing potential, than had they been told what you thought was their problem. This is the reason that questions play such an important role, because although one's ego finds it tempting to reveal all that you know about them from their feet, it can be an unwise game for you to play.

The role of questioning

The word "question" comes from the French *questionner*, meaning to seek. When we ask questions, we allow the person whose feet we are examining, to seek their own answers to the problem. Simple questions such as "How do you feel about your feet?" can reveal a great deal to the client when their answer is repeated back to them, this time in relation to themselves and not their feet.

For example, the other day a woman's answer to that question was "I used to love my feet, they were so beautiful. Now, they look old and wrinkled and two of the toes are twisted. It also hurts to walk on them. I dislike them so much now that I keep them covered. I feel ashamed of what has become of them." From this statement the woman was able to see how much she had come to dislike not only her feet, but also herself. Consequently, she had removed herself from close relationships, fearing that people would reject what they saw. This made life extremely painful for her and she compensated for her anguish by eating, making her feel even worse about herself. Had I not asked this question and jumped straight into my insights, this valuable realization might have been lost.

So the point is keep asking questions. Is it painful? How long has that been there? Do you feel your ideas are being battered down? Are you feeling fed up? Is there a man whose behaviour makes you feel angry? Are you feeling very afraid and vulnerable now? Tell me about your childhood - were you very strictly brought up? And so on. Then your friend or client can feel in control of what is happening, and you just provide a safe, contained space for their process to take place. Often people will say no to a suggestion on your part. Respect that, even if you feel they are in denial. That is their perogative and we have no right to push them beyond where they want to go.

Compassion

Can I see another's woe,
And not be in sorrow too?
Can I see another's grief'
And not seek for kind relief?
William Blake.[3]

Compassion means to suffer with someone. When we have compassion for another, we feel the pain of the path they have walked. Their pain becomes our pain. To be in the presence of someone, with deep compassion, is to have total non-judgmental acceptance and understanding of the problems they are facing. It is as if love fills up the spaces, which have become depleted in them, and in so doing, gives them the strength to continue on their journey. If you want to walk a spiritual path, just giving someone unconditional love, even if only for a few moments a day, is worth far more than a hundred workshops and self-development courses.

I once heard of a healer who did nothing but sit quietly with you on a lovely old bench in her garden, whilst holding your hand. Such was the depth of her compassion, that much healing took place. To feel completely accepted and loved seems such a small thing, yet so few people ever experience it in life. It is the basis of all we yearn for. Baby mice kept in cages and given the option of a nest with warm fur or a nest with milk, were found starved to death snuggled against the fur.

This need for unconditional acceptance or compassion then is at the core of our being, motivating much of our unconscious behaviour. However, in order to be able to give this compassion to others, we need to be able to give it to ourselves, which most of us find hard to do. We believe that it's noble to martyr ourselves by ignoring our own needs and suffer for others; but we miss the point. To be in balance we first need to have total love and acceptance for ourselves or else we cannot truly give to others. By denying our own needs, we demonstrate to ourselves a lack of compassion. So many healers, both allopathic and holistic, give and give to the point of burnout, often experiencing huge resentment when their own need for help are unmet. Working to the detriment of our own health is not showing compassion for ourselves. How then can we be truly compassionate to those we serve?

To practice compassion, allow yourself a few minutes of quiet time. Visualize energy flowing through your crown, into your head and down into your heart. Enjoy the feeling of warmth as your heart "lights up." Then visualize this warm light bathing your entire body flowing from the heart and going to any spaces where you may have aches or pain. Only when you have absorbed this warm light completely and feel totally fulfilled, start visualizing this light flowing from your heart and out into the world, surrounding and nurturing family, friends, colleagues, those in need, places, cities, countries, animals, the earth etc. Visualize this beautiful, light energy, flowing from your heart for as long as it feels right for you. This is a simple but very valuable and effective exercise in giving to yourself and others.

Now that your cup is full, you are ready to give to those who need attention.

Listening

There is an old saying that conveys the sense that we have been given two ears and one mouth for a reason. Obviously, the lesson is that we need to listen twice as much as we need to speak. Often simply listening to someone speak about events in their lives that have caused them pain, is sufficient to bring about huge transformation. I have spent many sessions with people who reveal aspects of their lives that have remained hidden for many, many years. The burden of carrying these issues has taken its toll. Simply to have another bear witness and share empathetically with your pain, goes very far along the road to healing it.

A young woman whose husband had rejected her sexually; an elderly man who had been accused of rape twenty years earlier and had never revealed this, or hating a sibling for forcing you to live in their shadow... we all have issues which burden us. We may feel so ashamed of these incidents or events that we carry them with us with each painful step we take.

One of the things I have learnt is that friends are there to offer us advice; counselors are there not to. None of the people I have just mentioned needed me to solve their problems. It would be egotistical in the extreme to believe I could in any case. Rather, they simply needed a safe space to let go of some of their burdens, and in doing so forgive themselves or those who had hurt them.

So listen, listen, *listen*. If you are busy thinking about your response, you may just miss a vital clue that might help the person. Very often mirroring back what they have said is a great way to help them help themselves. For example, someone may say:

"I really am angry with John for breaking up our marriage and for how abusive he was to me." You might respond, "I can understand that you are very angry with John both for breaking up your marriage and being abusive to you." "Yes, it was awful. I can't believe I allowed him to do what he did." Your response might be, "It sounds pretty awful, and I guess we all look back at our lives and get angry and regret what has happened." So the dialogue will continue as the client starts to unravel some of the tangle that has crept into their lives.

We lead such hectic lives and seldom find time for each other. It is a huge luxury just to have someone listen with complete attention to what you have to say. Remember this when you look at someone's feet. Another aspect in life, which is particularly visible when we work closely with someone, is that his or her issues will very often mirror our own. Much of what is in them is also in us, even if our experience of the situation may have been very different. After I lost my first baby, I was often put in situations with others who were dealing with loss. As I witnessed their pain, bravery and healing, so I too experienced my own healing and came to realisations that would not have been possible if I had not seen them as me and vice versa. Someone may be experiencing a physical loss of a job, while your loss may be more emotional, but the principles remain the same. They are your mirrors, just as you are theirs.

Remember also that the insights in this book are a guide only. I, and those who assist me, most certainly do not have all the answers. Jumping to conclusions can be as dangerous as jumping off a cliff!

To sum up then:

- Seeing into someone's soul is sacred. Treat it that way.
- Merely assist your clients to find their own answers.
- Get rid of your ego and the need to be right.
- Ban judgment.
- Listen, listen, *listen*.
- Don't give advice – give your clients the power to discover their own solutions.
- Have compassion for both you and your client.

SECTION 2

CONTENTS

SECTION II

Aspects of the Feet

From amputated toes to webbed toes and everything in between!

Amputated Toes

KEY ISSUES

Completely removed from or cut off from your own thoughts and ideas (that relate to the specific toe).

ORIGIN OF THE WORD

Originally, the word 'amputate' referred to the pruning back of trees or bushes. In a sense if a toe is cut off, our potential for growth in this area, is also cut-back, simply because if the toe is *cut-off*, the ability to draw in concepts/ideas/thoughts into the chakra concerned may be limited. However, the good news is that the aura or astral body of the missing toe, because it was there at birth, will still be visible to an aura reader, which means that although the toe is lost in the physical world, in the astral or energetic world, its potential remains.

LOSS OF BABY TOE

The baby toe relates to ideas or beliefs upheld by our society, religion or family. They also relate to our feelings of security within our family/society/religious group. If we decide to move away from the belief systems of any of these groups, it is seldom met with appreciation. (Imagine telling your fundamentalist Christian parents that you were embracing Buddhism!) If the event has been extremely dramatic or traumatic, we could find ourselves cut off from all the beliefs that we grew up with or, subconsciously, we could want to cut ourselves off from our family.

LOSS OF FOURTH TOE

The fourth toe relates to our one–on-one relationships and our beliefs regarding them, as well as to money and sex. To suffer an amputation then is to suffer the loss of one's understanding regarding how a relationship, money or sex, should be. We also may feel cutoff from our feelings, or unable to express them. When we cannot express how we feel to someone else, it affects our relationships. We cannot know someone deeply if they cannot communicate their feelings. Alternatively, we may battle to form our own ideas or beliefs, or may feel cutoff from pleasure. We may want to subconsciously cut ourselves off from a relationship with either a male or female (mother or father) depending on the foot concerned.

LOSS OF THIRD TOE

Loss of the **third toe** may cut us off from relating to ourselves and our anger. We may have no idea how we should respond to situations or ideas about how we can change. We may also not want to relate to aspects of ourselves.

LOSS OF SECOND TOE

When the **second toe** is amputated, we may feel removed from thoughts on love or have problems relating in love, both to ourselves and to others. We may subconsciously wish to remove ourselves from, say, a toxic marriage.

LOSS OF BIG TOE

The **big toe** is the most serious physical loss, because without it, balance is harder. We may feel cut off from our connection to God, or struggle to access new ideas and thoughts. We may wish to completely sever our old way of thinking regarding our religious beliefs. It may also refer to intellectual concepts that we no longer wish to accept.

For additional information on a specific toe or lack thereof, see Chapter Two. Also be aware of which foot the amputation is on: – i.e. right foot = male/past beliefs and left foot = female/present or current issues.

CASE STUDY

(In this study, because the child was very young, not much emotional input could be obtained. However, the events subsequent to the amputation proved interesting in their progression and so I have included them. Note: All studies are case specific. However, this does not mean that another person with a similar toe amputated will necessarily follow the same physical progression.)

A toddler had amputated her toe by pulling on the electrical cord of a heavy, ribbed, oil heater, causing the heater to topple over and smash onto the tiled floor. As it did so, it fell much like a guillotine onto her foot, amputating her fourth toe and cutting the foot between the second and third toe.

The only connection left between the toe and the foot was one small vein. Her mother picked up the toe, wrapped it in ice and drove the traumatized child to the hospital.

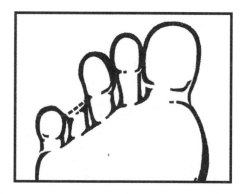

Fig. 34 · Amputated toe

The toe was joined to the foot with a thin piece of wire inserted into the bone of the toe and foot. The one vein still joining them managed to pump enough blood to the toe to sustain part of it. The top of the toe, however, fell away when the first bandage was removed. The shock to the child was such that she had a convulsion shortly afterwards and then lost consciousness. Follow-up brain tests revealed nothing abnormal and although doctors at the time would not link the two events, in homeopathy the link between a seizure following an amputation is known and acknowledged. (There is even a specific remedy for it.)

The lost aspect of the toe was on the right foot, indicating issues either with a male (in this case, because of her young age, it was most likely to be her father) her own masculine aspects, or issues from the past. It could also relate to past life issues, i.e. perhaps she had karmic past life issues in connection with her father. It must be noted that the child was not an easy baby to raise and this resulted in the father feeling some resentment towards the child and these feelings drove a wedge between him and his wife.

It is interesting that this amputation of the top of the toe, which relates to the head, is caused by a disturbance in the brainwave transmission. The brain is situated in the area where the toe was lost. By severing the head of the toe, it is likely then that this produced a mirror in the brain, which triggered the fit.

FURTHER DEVELOPMENTS

Subsequently the child developed asthma a year later and, at the age of six, Bell's Palsy.

Asthma relates to fear, trust issues, feeling smothered or needing to smother an emotional upset. The inner rhythm of giving and receiving is disturbed so that the asthmatic has to gasp to get air and then battles to expel it. Taking in air becomes a frantic need and with it there is a reluctance to let it go. This indicates how needy the asthma sufferer is for love and attention. He or she holds onto what they have and yet this threatens to suffocate them.

Trust is also an issue. Air is abundant, yet the asthma sufferer unconsciously feels a lack of it. They don't trust the world to provide for them. The world becomes a threatening place, where anything from dust, to grass, to cats' hair, is seen as a threat. He or she is afraid to embrace life: - to breathe it in deeply. The problem, if untreated, can lead to a barrel-type of chest, which indicates the sufferer is literally trying to puff his/her chest out to mask feelings of inadequacy. Because it affects their fourth chakra it indicates a longing for love, which they try to breathe in, yet are afraid when it comes to giving.

Palsy also relates to fear and anxiety and not being able to express feelings. (The toe amputated relates to feelings.) Like the story of the little boy who made horrible faces and whose face became stuck in a grimace when the wind blew, so in Palsy (which incidentally can be physically brought on by exposure to icy wind as was so in this case), her "stuck" face emphasized that she was *frozen with fear*. Although appearing unconcerned at attending the new school, her physical reactions revealed otherwise. Having this toe amputated, which is symbolic of expressing feelings and relationships, indicated that there was a link between the two events and that the palsy was a visible form of the inner fear that she was unable to express.

This difficulty with relating her feelings to others and feeling disconnected to those close to her, understandably had this child not trusting that she would receive love unconditionally. Both the palsy and the asthma indicate this child's mistrust and fear of life. Like many asthmatics, she swung from puffing her chest out in exaggerated importance, in an attempt to control relationships, to its opposite expression of inadequacy and attempting to deal with her smallness (she was the youngest child in the family).

Given that it was the second chakra, it would indicate that the child felt cut off from not only her own feelings, but from the feelings of others. With the toe gone, understanding relationships and their functioning was hard. The child felt cut off from her father, who seemed emotionally and often physically, absent for much of her childhood.

At times the neck of the toe would crack open and bleed, because of the odd shape of the toe, indicating how painful and wounded communication and expression had become. The nail grew, but only a very small part of it, leaving the toe vulnerable and exposed, just as the child felt in relationships. The way she attempted to control this world that felt so uncertain, was to try to dominate it with her needs. (Asthmatics can't go to certain places that may put them at risk; they have to have special bedding, must avoid areas where people smoke etc. Through this they exert a certain control over the family who must conform to their needs.)

This child also had a hugely swollen heart area, indicating how much emotion was bottled up inside, unable to be expressed. By understanding the child's nature, the parents were encouraged to find ways for the child to communicate her feelings. Gently asking how the child was feeling after a certain event, opened the door for a flow of communication. Art was helpful in this process, although the child was resistant at first. The toe itself would not grow back, but by building the child's trust and self-confidence, she would learn to breathe for herself and then would be able to build solid, trusting relationships with others.

Ankle Sprains and Breaks

KEY ISSUES
Strain in changing/moving ahead. Unable to go with the flow. Collapsing with guilt and pressure. Inflexible.

PHYSICAL CAUSES
Without our feet, we could not move forward in our lives. We spend hours on our feet every day, taking several thousand steps, each of which puts a load equivalent to two to three times one's body weight on them. The ankle is the prime connecting support for the body and bears the brunt of this force. It's not surprising then that the ankle comes under so much pressure, both physically and emotionally. Ankles are particularly vulnerable, because they are much thinner than the rest of the leg, yet carry the same weight.

Most ankle injuries usually occur on the outside (lateral side) of the ankle. An ankle sprain can be extremely painful, causing bruising and tenderness. Mild sprains can be treated with RICE (Rest, Ice, Compression and Elevation). The pain usually disappears in a few days.

ORIGIN OF THE WORDS AND THEIR RELEVANCE
The word ankle comes from *ank,* meaning to bend or twist. The ankles themselves represent our flexibility in life and, as we have seen, our support and mobility. When we strain or sprain an ankle, we are collapsing from the pressure of having to move forward in life. Alternatively, we may feel unable to move ahead, bending to internal or external pressure not to change. Once we have sprained our ankle, it is often bound up tightly and becomes inflexible and we can't move.

EMOTIONAL CAUSES
As stated, the majority of injuries are on the external side of the ankle, affecting the pelvis, hips and legs, as mirrored on the feet.

All these bones are essential in allowing us to move forward. If we feel pressured to move forward and yet *dig our heels in*, the resulting push/pull situation creates a tension between a need to move forward and because of fear, a resistance to do so. Under the strain the ankles collapse. The hips also relate to our sexuality, while our pelvis relates to birthing issues and to our mothers who birthed us. If the strain affects this corresponding area on our ankles, around the outside protruding

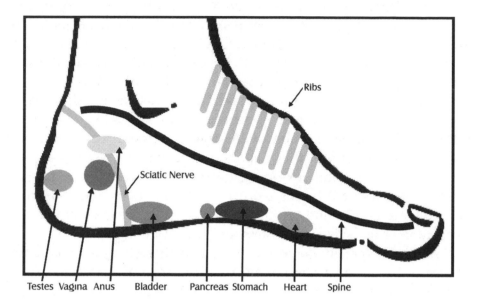

Testes Vagina Anus   Bladder   Pancreas Stomach   Heart   Spine

Fig. 35 · Side of feet - This shows how the organs on underside of feet wrap round onto the side of the foot.

anklebone, then we could look at where there is strain involved with moving either physically or emotionally away from our mothers.

The only time I ever sprained an ankle was when I left home for the first time to go on holiday with a boyfriend. My subsequent sprained left ankle (present, female side) in the area of the hip in the ankle (mother), revealed the fear and strain I had in breaking away from home. Obviously, a break rather than a sprain would cause a far more serious emotional reaction in having to overcome our rigidity and resistance. Being immobile and having to remain lying or sitting while the ankle healed, would also mirror that we may have a problem *standing up* to others.

CASE STUDY

In an interesting case involving just these emotions, I heard of a young man who was the only son of a divorced mother. She had been living alone for many years, and had suffered bouts of depression, so looked to her son for support. Because she felt insecure, she was extremely controlling, of life in general and of her son in particular. He had resisted this, first by enlisting in the army and then later by going to study in a faraway town. There, after a brief period of wild student exploits, he formed a steady relationship. For the first few holidays he either did not go home, or went alone to stay with his mother. After the relationship had lasted a year, he took his girlfriend to holiday with his family.

Three years into the relationship, he decided to take his girlfriend on holiday alone to stay at a small guesthouse at the sea, rather than participate in the usual family holiday. As the guesthouse was only a few hours drive from his mother, he agreed to spend two days with her initially. Once at his mother's home, however, the man found himself increasingly pressured by his mother to remain there. She seemed to have forgotten the boundary lines he had initially negotiated for a two-day stay and she increased the pressure as time went by.

Caught between his own needs, that of his girlfriend's and the desires of his mother, the young man did not know which way to turn. He wanted to move forward and establish his independence and yet a history of complying with his mother's wishes, stopped him. This caused the man a huge emotional strain, and far from being relaxed, he found himself caught in an emotionally manipulative trap. Eventually he plucked up the courage to take a stand, go against his mother's wishes and he did *make the break*, much to his mother's anger.

Relieved at having fought and won his independence, he set out to enjoy himself. After finding the guest house and settling in, he set out to kite-board in the surf. The exhilaration was extreme as he flew from one wave peak to the next, twisting turning and gliding with masterful control. Now he felt the full freedom his courageous stance had allowed. For the first time in his life he was not dependent on his mother for finance (he had a job) and revelled in his personal growth.

However, half an hour into his first sail, he took off from a wave and landed badly, completely snapping his left ankle, to the extent that he actually heard the crack. Drifting helplessly in the surf, he was eventually found by a paddle-skier, who dragged him to shore, in a rescue that took the better part of an hour. Once at the hospital, metal plates and screws had to be inserted in order to support the ankle. On hearing of his accident his mother, in spite of his protests, came down to see him and stayed with him during his convalescence. Now he was not only helpless, but at the mercy of those who looked after him. It was a hard lesson in independence.

This interesting case involves all the aspects covered: mother issues, strain in moving forward, guilt, collapse, rigidity and pressure, both from his mother, who refused to accept the change in her son's relationship towards her and from his girlfriend to *take a stand*. Having done so, the strain was too much to bear, and his left (female/present) ankle, snapped from the pressure, making moving forward impossible.

Because he felt so guilty about going against the wishes of his mother, a saboteur archetype developed in him – he did not feel he deserved to be happy, which resulted in the accident, after which he was unable to enjoy the pleasures he had planned. He now found himself not only wounded but completely subjected to the attentions of his mother whom he had stood up against.

By understanding the emotional aspect of what had occurred, he was able to come to terms not only with the experience but with himself and the need to establish his independence more.

HEALING

If there are ankle problems, then we need to ask ourselves where we are under pressure to change or move forward. Are you finding it a strain to stand up for yourself? If it is the left ankle look at female issues within yourself or females that you may think are influencing you to feel this way. If it is the right ankle look at men and your male issues. Are you carrying guilt about the situation? Are you feeling pressurized to move and are resisting doing so? Do you feel you deserve the right to enjoy yourself? Do you just need to change direction? Do you feel unsupported in change? Are you rigidly holding onto your present situation? Are you struggling to remain flexible?

If the answer to any of these questions is "Yes," then ask yourself how it is serving you to remain where you are physically, emotionally or mentally. Do you really want to remain there? What would your life be like if you did not have this issue? If it were better or freer, why would you want to hold on to this way of thinking/feeling/being? Maybe its time to let it go – to move ahead trusting in the process of life and the Divine to assist you on the next stage of your journey.

Arthritis in the Feet

KEY ISSUES

Difficulty with change, resentment, repressed anger, rigidity, control issues, judgmental attitudes, needing approval from others.

ORIGIN OF THE WORD

Artho means joint and *itis* means inflammation. While arthritis affects many parts of the body, it frequently affects the feet.

PHYSICAL CAUSES

The most common of the approximately 38 types of arthritis is osteoarthritis, where the cartilage of the joints degenerates or tears away. Old age, excessive weight, ill-fitting shoes and trauma (injury) are its most common causes. The feet are frequently affected and movement can become extremely painful.

Approximately 350 million people in the world suffer from have arthritis. Nearly one in three adults in the United States are affected (roughly 66 million people,) according to 2005 statistics of the Arthritis Foundation, including over a quarter million children! It is also the leading cause of disability in America for people over the age of 15. Surprisingly, more than half of those with arthritis are under 65 years of age, of which approximately 60% are women.[1]

We require our feet to walk or move ahead in life. The joints and the limbs they serve allow the movement to be fluid. Where there is stiffness or pain, this movement becomes difficult, indicating that the ability to change may be harder for someone with arthritic feet. The inflammation that accompanies this movement shows the degree of anger or resentment involved when life forces one to move.

EMOTIONAL CAUSES

The lack of fluid in the joints implies that our inflamed (fire) thoughts are drying us up (water) emotionally. We can see then that there is an imbalance between the fiery (masculine principle) and watery (female principle) aspects of ourselves. This we can interpret as the desire to do and be expansive and move ahead, versus the desire to contract, be passive and resist change. The resulting tension that builds up between the two aspects within us causes this imbalance. Depending on which foot is the most affected (right foot = past issues and the masculine principle;

left foot = the feminine principle, present issues) this will show us which aspects are more dominant.

Because we resist change in our way of thinking, our thoughts and bones become calcified and wear away both our bones and our minds. We may attempt to control the speed of change, as well as trying to control those around us as part of this process. The frustration or bitterness that builds up when others fail to comply can be seen in the inflammation of the joints. We may feel we are victims to their behaviour and feel angry that they do not meet our needs. We may also want to change and dislike ourselves for not doing so. We may want to go with the flow, be spontaneous and live in the moment, but our fear and resistance to change has us trying to control the rate of change, lacking spontaneity and dwelling on past issues. We may find ourselves harshly critical of our own behaviour and the behaviour of others. We may both need and want attention and love, and yet find it so hard to receive. We may be needy of others and resent them (and ourselves) for our need.

(It's interesting that two of the main things that an arthritic sufferer must not indulge in are wine and tomatoes. Tomatoes have sometimes been called the "Fruits of Love," while wine has long been associated with seduction and love, as in Bacchus, the god of drunken revelry and sexual pleasure. Therefore, even in what they eat or drink, arthritics are restricted from letting go and experiencing the love they desire.)

CASE STUDY

Stephanie had arthritis in the big toe of her left foot as well as in both hands. (The right hand was worse than the left hand.) She ran an agency that imports car parts. Successful and career orientated, she still works in spite of being in her sixties. She divorced her first husband; the second had died some years before and she again had remarried. Although her third husband was able to support her, she wanted to ensure her financial independence and so continued to work.

She was proud of her long blonde hair and good looks, maintaining herself with regular workouts at the gym and eating a healthy diet. In complete opposition to this, she smoked and had a drinking problem resulting in wild binges followed by periods of teetotalism. (In other words she was an alcoholic.) She mentioned that her job had always put her under stress and believed that it was this stress that was causing her arthritis. She had come to believe that stress was simply part of life.

Further enquiry revealed that the stress was specifically caused by anger that had flared up inside her and that she was unable to express. Her husband was prone to mood swings and she complied each time he changed a plan, with no visible show of anger. For instance, she would prepare supper and he would announce that they should go out instead. Or he would plan a quiet evening at home and then arrive home with a group of hungry friends. She did not try to deal with problems but rather avoided them by drinking. This suppression of aggression is typical of the fiery nature of arthritis and the physical inflammation that it causes.

Much of this client's anger or frustration arose from having to conform to her husband's beliefs and ideas (what the big toe represents), which imposed limitations on her. These beliefs related more to her female side that had to conform to the male in her life. Hence the occurrence of the arthritis in her left (female) side, as it was her female side that felt these limitations.

As well as having to meet the changing needs of her husband, she spoke about having to meet the needs of the company she ran, often in opposition to her own needs. She mentioned that she was not a martyr, yet much of her behaviour indicated otherwise; she saw this more as a need to be needed, rather than a sacrifice. Once again the arthritic theme of rigid beliefs, neediness and repressed anger were at play. Like many arthritic sufferers, my client's history revealed a life of excessive activity. From working tirelessly at home and in the office, exercising regularly at the gym, and also entertaining clients, she was constantly active. Her drinking was an attempt to drown or water down her fire/anger about having to do these things. (She had spoken of drinking to stave off depression). She had sacrificed her own needs tirelessly for the sake of others. Now this life of stressful activity was causing an opposite reaction by creating rigidity and immobility. As in all imbalances, the body was seeking balance.

Yet whilst being active physically, her thoughts remained rigid . Arthritic sufferers are often extremely conscientious to the point of perfectionism (which often shows up as high arches and rigid, visible tendons on the top of the foot). This need to be perfect often comes at the expense of sacrificing our own needs and desires, in order to please others. This again leads to a repressed anger, which is masked by over-politeness or exaggerated helpfulness and may sometimes lead to depression.

In examining repressed anger further, some interesting symbology appears. The hands are how we give and receive, and with arthritis the hands tend to close up, much like a boxer's fist. The person then finds it hard to open up and receive. In turn they become closed to receiving input from others and struggle to give of themselves - not of their time or labour, but of their emotional selves. A fist is also a symbol of aggression, as in having a *clenched fist*. My client's clenched hands were an indication of the repressed aggression that she harboured and could not release. The fiery inflammation in her joints also symbolized her repressed anger. The pain she felt was the pain that deep down she would like to have inflicted upon those whom she served and whose approval she sought by sacrificing her own needs.

This was clearly demonstrated by the pain she was currently experiencing in her toe which had *flared* up over the weekend. She had dutifully entertained some clients for the weekend in spite of resenting having to do so. To add *fuel to her fire*, one client in particular was not appreciative of the experience. This enraged her, but as usual she repressed her anger and resentment. Thus the pain she felt in her foot was the pain she would rather have directed at the client. In restraining herself from saying anything, she had redirected her hostility towards herself.

Often the arthritic sufferer feels guilty for feeling aggressive and to compensate, seeks to be of service to others, which in turn causes more resentment - and so the cycle continues.

Acid is a fiery element and arthritic sufferers usually have very acidic systems, which is another sign of the fire or anger they carry. Depressive moods are another sign of repressed aggression. Depression comes from the root word in Latin *deprimo*, which means to press down. What we press down or suppress, must at some point be released or expressed. The repressed aggression may lead to depression – the fire of anger, out of balance, swings into the opposite wateriness of depression.

Although she did acknowledge her needs and emotions regarding security issues, the approval of others, her frustration at meeting the needs of others and difficulty in receiving, my client was unwilling to explore these emotions and the more questions I asked and the closer she got to finding the answers, the greater her resistance to the process became. I fully accepted her position, realizing that the habits of sixty years cannot be changed in one session and that change is not something any of us, particularly those with rigidity problems, embrace.

I do hope though that some of our discussion may have sparked some interest and that she may be inclined to take the process further at some stage. Doing so could free her up to experience more freedom and less pain in the years ahead.

HEALING: CONVENTIONAL HEALING

There are many allopathic medications that have been developed to alleviate the pain and progress of arthritis. Homeopathic remedies have also been helpful in many cases, as have a wide range of remedies including selenium, evening primrose oil, copper bracelets, avocados, reflexology, massage, Reiki and also by avoiding tobacco, tomatoes, potatoes and peppers.

EMOTIONAL HEALING

We need to look at freeing ourselves up and here modalities where fluidity in the body is practiced, such as yoga, may be useful. We also need to find ways to give to and nurture ourselves; to let go of the past, which no longer serves us; and ask the question why, when it makes us so unhappy, do we refuse to forgive or change. We need to ask ourselves what events, situations and pain we are holding onto. What would we need to do to move freely and let go and let God? How does it serve us *not* to do this?

We need to understand that all the judgments and fault finding we have about other people, are really judgments we have about ourselves. To heal this wound we need to start appreciating the positive aspects of what we are and not dwell on what we are not. We need to work on trusting the process of life, to see the beauty and love inside ourselves and other people, to have compassion for our struggles in life and to appreciate the excitement of exploring the unknown. It is not an easy path to walk, as our feet show, but letting go of the past will lighten our load.

Athlete's Foot and Fungus Problems

KEY ISSUES
Sadness and hurt at needing or wanting the approval and recognition of others for our efforts, thoughts or ideas and not receiving the recognition we crave.

PHYSICAL CAUSES
Athlete's Foot typically affects the skin on the feet between any of the last four toes. In extreme cases, it can affect the toenails, which untreated can become thick and distorted. It can also spread, through contact, to other parts of the body such as the groin or underarms. It is thought to be transferred by walking on floors that are moist, such as in gyms, public showers, around swimming pools, saunas or through contact with infected peoples' towels or shoes.

Athlete's Foot thrives in damp conditions. Bacterial infection may result as a secondary infection, worsening the symptoms and making it more difficult to cure. As it is a fungal infection, and the feet are naturally moist due to perspiration, Athlete's Foot can be very hard to treat.

ORIGIN OF WORDS
To determine its emotional symbology, we must look at the nature of a fungus, as well as the symbol of the toes where the fungus most commonly manifests. The word fungus comes from the Greek word *spongos*. From this word we derive the word *sponge*, as well as *fungus*. The verb sponge means to live off another, much the same as any species in nature, which lives in a parasitic manner. Currently saying someone is *sponging off* someone else means they exist parasitically on the welfare and charity of another (although in past interpretations, the victim was the sponge from which others squeezed the life essence). The reference to an athlete is also interesting. On a physical level, its association is obviously because athletes spend time in gyms and locker rooms, where the fungus purportedly is spread. The word athlete comes from the verb *athlein*, meaning to compete for a prize. When we compete for a prize, we are seeking to win approval from another – some reward for our efforts. Not receiving the prize or praise makes us sore and hurt.

EMOTIONAL CAUSES

When we find Athlete's Foot on our feet we need to examine where we are being squeezed or sucked dry by another whose approval we require. Are others being parasitic, emotionally or physically in our lives, or taking advantage of our kind nature? As the most common occurrence of Athletes Foot is between and underneath the toes (an area that relates to our thinking as well as expressing our thoughts) our need for recognition usually relates to wanting our ideas and thoughts acknowledged.

When waiting to see how my first book, *Healing Habits* would be accepted, I frequently found myself with Athlete's Foot. Would my ideas about the emotional causes of various habits presented in the book be met with scorn or praise? Had I put too much pressure on myself to get the book written, while coping with children and my normal work? How would I feel if the book was rejected, or would I win the prize of approval? My lesson was in learning to let go of the attachment to either outcome.

As the skin peels and cracks it becomes raw and painful. Likewise we need to look at where we feel sore, exposed and raw. The cut-like crevices that form between the toes also indicate feeling *cut up* about the situation, as well as removed or cut off from those whom we see as withholding praise or who seem to be using us. As mentioned previously, the fungus can only live in a moist environment and moisture denotes feelings and tears. Therefore, it would appear that Athlete's Foot thrives in a highly-charged emotional environment.

The toes represent our thoughts and the details in our lives. If others drain our thoughts, or us, we may become sore, resentful and pained. We may feel as if we are cracking up in certain areas. Because the infection also often spreads to the top of the underside of the foot, just beneath the toes where the heart chakra is located, feelings of lack of acceptance, recognition, or of being used, may be causing us considerable grief. In addition, the skin peels off, implying layers of emotional issues being peeled away to expose the raw hurt and pain. Also the redness indicates there may be anger involved as well.

When the toenails thicken, it shows us we have developed an additional shield or protection against the hurt we feel at not being acknowledged, or being sponged off.

By understanding what each toe represents, and examining between which toes the fungus has manifested, we can arrive at an even more accurate picture of where our dis-ease originated.

Athlete's Foot is found most commonly under or between the two smallest toes. This is not coincidental, but rather because Athlete's Foot demonstrates the person's need for approval, which requires other individuals, families or corporations to feed it. Hence it falls under the toes relating to families, groups of people for instance at church, or with whom we work and in our one-on-one relationships. If the middle toe is involved, then it would also include our relationship to ourselves. Sometimes we are our own worst enemies in withholding approval of ourselves. We continue to draw or sponge from our resources without recognizing our achievements.

Diabetes can sometimes cause a sore that may appear to be a bad form of Athlete's Foot. If in any doubt, contact your doctor.

Athlete's Foot found between the second and third toes

(fourth/ third chakra issues) Relates to having ideas that affect our self-esteem and self-acceptance whilst not recognizing our own ideas and achievements. Can also relate to ideas on intimacy or love, where we feel we are being drained or used.

Athlete's Foot found between third and fourth toes

(third/second chakra issues) Relates to our thoughts about our self-esteem, personal integrity, relationships with others and how we feel when we don't receive acknowledgement, or when others use us. It can also be linked to what is galling us, or making us bitter. Money can also be an issue. Is someone draining our financial resources by using our concepts or ideas? Do we want recognition for our ideas from a partner who is withholding it? Are we upset when we don't appear to be accepted by others?

Athlete's Foot found between fourth and baby toes

(second/first chakra issues) Relates to large groups of people or corporations, as well as families, and the individuals in them. Is the company we work for draining us intellectually? Do we feel our family is sponging off us? Is this affecting our security? Are we looking for recognition of our achievements from our colleagues, or family and upset because this is not forthcoming?

CASE STUDY

One client I saw had a fungal develop on the foot in the area of the solar plexus and adrenal gland which was an angry red circle, the size of a large coin and was both painful and inflamed. My client(let's call him Allan) had been to see a doctor who suspected that it was some kind of infection from an STD (sexually transmitted disease). Allan was horrified, as he had not been unfaithful to his wife, and so disagreed with the doctor's diagnosis. However, none of the creams prescribed cleared up the angry flaking area.

As I learned more about Allan, I discovered he had a very high pressure job in marketing and lived in constant fear of not achieving the goals set for him by management. He was by nature a gentle artistic man, wholly unsuited for the aggressive, demanding world of his chosen career. He had a superb mind and was highly creative, yet his concepts seldom received recognition from his superiors. During the time he had the fungus (a later diagnosis indicated that's what it was), a younger man had been employed in a position senior to my client. This young man never missed an opportunity to pull rank and make Allan feel inadequate and inferior. The problem was, however, that Allan had all the ideas which his superior could not even begin to imagine. Consequently, Allan's ideas were constantly being poached and dressed up to look as if they had been those of his superior. Unwilling by nature to enter into conflict, Allan had accepted this situation for the sake of maintaining his job.

It was during this period of his life that the red fungus wheel appeared on his right foot. Being in the area of the solar plexus, it indicated his anger at this dishonest representation of his work. The fungus had invaded his boundaries, just as his new boss was doing. As the fungus also covered the adrenal glands, this also showed that Allan was very afraid he might lose his job (security first chakra) if he threatened to reveal the true nature of what was happening. As layer after layer of skin peeled away, he felt more and more vulnerable and pained by the situation. His defenses were being *eaten away*.

Once able to realize why he had developed this fungus, it gradually disappeared and Allan began very gingerly to confront his superior. As luck would have it, the entire company was then sold and the younger man was one of the casualties in the takeover. Allan remained at work assuming a more senior position and the fungus did not return while I was still in contact with him. I heard later he had left the field of marketing.

HEALING

In order to heal Athlete's Foot, we have to let go of the need for accept-ance and approval from others. As long as we continue to seek recogni-tion and emotional reward from others, we put ourselves in a position of constantly being manipulated or drained by them. As long as we allow it, they will continue to draw and sponge off us; the hard part is that we need to accept that it is *our* need for approval which has created the situation. Once we can accept that, we can work at trusting our-selves to move forward with our ideas, irrespective of what others think. We can acknowledge the pain and hurt we feel and choose to let it go. Then we have to work at giving approval to ourselves and acknowledge our own accomplishments without the need for recognition by others.

Blisters

KEY ISSUES
Friction. Resistance to the friction. Build-up of emotions around a situation.

PHYSICAL CAUSES
Go for a 10km hike in a new pair of boots and the chances are you will develop at least one blister, simply because the shoes rubbing up against your foot cause friction, which results in the watery fluid buildup under the skin. That's the physical reason for getting a blister. The emotional one mirrors the physical, in that whenever there is water there are emotional issues; combine this with emotional friction and you have the root emotional cause of a blister, namely a build-up of emotions as a result of friction.

ORIGIN OF WORD
The word blister comes from *blyster* meaning to swell, which links to the build-up of friction and the residue of emotions that swell within us. We also speak about a *blistering attack* on something or someone, meaning the attack is so ferocious that it can cause us to erupt in emotion.

EMOTIONAL CAUSES
Someone or something has literally *rubbed you up the wrong way.* For there to be friction any schoolchild will tell you that there has to be resistance. As an advertisement for a motor oil goes, "The less the friction the further you go." The same could be said for our lives. The more friction we have, the more we hold ourselves back from growth, as our energy is all being channelled into the fiery fight. Being filled with fire causes the watery build-up, as we try to balance our fire with water. So where the blisters are, also points to where we are resisting what is happening. Heat can also cause a blister and here the interpretation would be the same - a build up of heat/anger at a situation but because there has not been friction, there may be less resistance on our part.

In the army blisters are common, as new recruits spend long and painful hours marching and drilling. Emotionally though it is an indication of how, through the discipline of daily life, they find they are being *rubbed up the wrong way.* There is constant friction as orders are given that the recruit may find unreasonable. However, he is unable to express his emotion, as doing so could result in placed in detention. So this emotion builds and forms blisters.

Where a blister occurs will give insight into what exactly is causing friction within us. If on the toes it may relate to resistance to another's ideas or someone else resisting our ideas. It could also mean our ideas are causing friction. If the blister is on the ball of the foot, it could mean there is resistance to another's feelings (or friction about the way they feel) which is affecting us and may be making us feel vulnerable. If the blister is on the heel, then it is likely there is friction with the family/work /religious group. Alternatively, there may be friction about issues making us afraid to move ahead, or from feelings of insecurity.

Ask yourself questions such as the following: Where is there friction in my life? Where am I resisting change? Who angers me? Am I expressing that anger honestly and clearly? What issues or person may be contributing to my emotional build-up?

CASE STUDY

Carrie's blisters were not the classic blister that appears as a result of a tight shoe after a long walk. Rather they were a series of about ten tiny blisters in a group on her right foot in the area of her solar plexus, under the second toe. While they were most likely caused by a fungal infection, the fact that they resembled blisters physically, prompted me to consider them as such.

I began by asking Carrie where she might be experiencing friction in her life. As the group of blisters was on her right foot only, I suggested that this friction might have to do with either a man, or her own inner male - or both. Carrie replied that she was experiencing a great deal of friction in her marriage and felt this was where the problem lay. That the blisters fell on the solar plexus (where we feel anger) and below the second toe (related to her heart/marriage) was also very relevant. The small pockets of fluid were indicative of the tears she had not allowed herself to cry. As the sole provider for their four children, (her husband had not worked for five years,) Carrie had every reason to feel anger. Like the blisters, the anger remained beneath the surface and was only expressed by small resistances, rather than in one big blow-up.

Her husband was into alternative therapies and by rejecting him, she had also rejected much of her own spiritual path, as his beliefs seemed to be at the core of their problems. Consequently, it did not surprise me that there was a big callus over her pituitary gland, as the pituitary gland is our inner sight and gateway to our spirituality, which, like the proverbial baby in the bathwater, she had tossed aside.

Her feet were very flaccid and showed very little life force which, given the long hard hours she worked both at the office, and at home, was not surprising when combined with the amount of energy the friction in the household was causing.

Large calluses around the heel also indicated her insecurity fears , which were very relevant, as the family was in debt. That the calluses were starting to crack showed just how much the situation was cracking her up. As for the fungal aspect, Carrie related strongly to my question asking if she was receiving any recognition for her efforts from her husband. (Not receiving recognition and allowing others to take advantage of us is part of the symbology of fungal infections.)

HEALING

Blisters heal in a relatively short time. Often when the blister pops and the fluid is released, we feel a physical relief. This same relief is mirrored emotionally when we express (as opposed to suppress) what we feel. Letting it all pour out can be healing in itself. In many cases though, the skin forms a callus after the blister has burst. We have released the pent-up emotion, but now we need to build a wall of protection around ourselves. As the skin peels off, we experience a gradually sloughing-off to do with the problem triggering the blisters. We have let it go. If, on the other hand, the blister becomes infected, this is an indication that the situation has become infested with poisonous feelings.

Bruises

KEY ISSUES

Over-sensitive. Feeling hurt and emotionally sore. Feeling beaten-up by life.

PHYSICAL CAUSES

When we get knocked or hit, our blood capillaries and blood vessels become damaged and blood drains into the tissues. The variety of colours that result are caused by the amount of blood and the contents of the actual blood cells themselves. People who bruise easily may either have fragile capillaries, or problems with the clotting mechanism in the body.

ORIGIN OF THE WORD

Bruise comes from the Old English *brysan* which means to crush and also from the Old French *bruisier*, meaning to break. As we shall see, those who bruise easily often feel crushed and broken by life itself, or by others.

EMOTIONAL CAUSES

People who bruise easily are more vulnerable to feeling hurt than other people. Usually being bruised on the feet involves having stepped down on something hard, or having pressure put onto that part of the foot by a hard object. The questions we would need to ask ourselves then are: What is hurting us and preventing us moving ahead? Are we so busy looking into the future, that we keep failing to see obstacles in the present? What makes it painful to move ahead? It often surprises me to see feet with bad bruising and the client has no recollection of how he or she got the bruises.

CASE STUDY

Sally seemed to float into the room. Tall and willowy, I felt an airy gentleness exude from her. It was not surprising to find that her feet had very small narrow heels (first chakra) and a wide top part, indicating that she was more involved with the airy than earthly realms chakra After massaging her feet, I asked her if she often felt disconnected, removed or floating above reality. She said that she did and she sometimes felt that she was a bit mad because she would often see this big 'presence' with whom she communicated.

She had a permanent bruise (a blue/red marking) on the underside of her small left toe, which had been there for as long as she could recall. As we spoke, it became apparent that her childhood had been far from happy. She was the illegitimate child of a prostitute and, unable to keep her child, given her lifestyle, the mother had organized for her daughter to be adopted when she was a few months old. Rejected by her real mother, the baby must have felt as if her roots had been destroyed. Her small heels (first chakra) made perfect sense given the feelings of abandonment she must have experienced (she mentioned not even knowing her birth date) and the lack of being able to bond or experience any connection to her birth mother.

Working on an intuitive feeling, I asked her whether she had ever suffered from an eating disorder. She replied she that she had. (I have found that people suffering from eating disorders also have poor bonding skills, and substance abuse is common in one or both parents.). When we are rejected by our mother and have bonding issues, we lack the ability to nurture ourselves adequately; consequently, eating disorders are likely and cause problems with obesity, or the opposite being underweight, Eating disorders disconnect us from our roots or physical bodies. Through tremendous courage and willpower, Sally had managed to overcome her eating problems and her drug dependence, and although struggling to establish a lasting loving relationship, she did find some security in her job.

She had been adopted by an elderly couple, which gave her life some sense of stability. In time, however, the couple's relationship deteriorated and they divorced, causing yet another upheaval in the Sally's life. An interesting aspect of this case was that her adoptive parents had changed her name completely from that given to her by her original mother. From numerology (the study of numbers and their influence on our lives) Sally discovered that in spite of her completely new name, the numerological value of both names was exactly the same, i.e. changing her parents had not altered her destiny.

We spoke about her childhood and the unhappiness she had experienced. She had pretty much got the whole package when it comes to childhood traumas, from being rejected, then adopted and then later abused.

I had noticed when she arrived that she was very apologetic about her feet and so I wasn't surprised to find that she had little self-esteem in spite of her attractive looks. (As mentioned earlier, not liking her feet indicated Sally disliked herself.)

If her mother's abandonment had been the cause of her first chakra wound, then her adopted family was the reason for her third chakra issues. She spoke of authoritative parents, abuse, manipulation etc. Looking at the blue/red bunions below her large toe, I asked her if all this had resulted in her trying desperately to please others at the expense of herself, which caused her both pain and anger. She agreed this was the case as she could not, even now, really accept compliments from others and constantly worried about not being good enough. We spoke then about the concept of never being able to enjoy the moment if we are constantly waiting to be good enough in the future.

She had big calluses on her heart, thyroid and pituitary reflexes. I explained calluses (and how they form from an emotional point of view) and that it was quite understandable that she might want to seal off her heart from hurt. As I worked on her pituitary reflex she mentioned being frustrated because she did not know what her purpose was in life. This was amazing as her calluses symbolized her block. We spoke about what we mean by our 'soul's purpose' and how it is often confused with what job we have. This led on to the callused thyroid which I felt showed she was so busy trying that she wasn't allowing herself the space to just simply be.

Her feet were very cold indicating a lack of joy and passion in life. When I asked her if this was true and she said it was but it depressed her to think of her life this way. We also then addressed the issue of fear, as this was showing up as a major problem in all areas of her life. She was afraid to express her real self for fear of not pleasing others; there was fear of failure; fear to change; fear of becoming an addict again, etc.; and the many criss-crossed lines in her instep also showed a confusion as to which direction in life to take.

Seeing large bags under all her toe-pads, I asked if she suffered from sinus or post-nasal drip and she said that she currently did.

To me, the bruise on her small toe symbolized all the pain and hurt that she had carried with her throughout her life. It also revealed feelings of being a victim of her circumstances. The redness was an indication of her anger towards the past events of her life and in particular towards her birth mother. It was as if life kept on beating her up.

I felt she needed to feel nurtured and have a connection to Mother Earth, so I suggested that she spend time in nature and allow herself to feel her connection to the earth. Eating wholesome, earthy type foods such as potatoes, and connecting to her body through aerobics, gardening and sports, would also help reestablish a connection to her physical self. I also suggested having massages as a way to feel nurtured.

Sometime later Sally told me she had reconnected with her birth mother, only to watch her die from Aids. However, a relationship was established and a number of past issues were released. Her toe represented the sore aspect of her family history that was always with her as she met each challenge life offered. And by counseling other drug users to assist in their rehabilitation, she was able to work through many of her own wounds, as well as become a valuable and much loved member of society.

HEALING
Bruises are red and black or blue in colour. Does this mean life is making you angry or you have the feeling that you are being beaten up by another? Does it feel as if you are being abused in some way? If so, you may understandably be feeling vulnerable and sore in this area. Are you being oversensitive? Do you hurt easily? Refer to Chapter Two for specific areas of your life where this may be occurring.

Bunions

KEY ISSUES
Reaching out for love. Trying hard. Desire for approval and perfectionism.

PHYSICAL CAUSES
Bunions are deformities or swellings caused by the bones at the base of the big toe angulating outwards on the inner side of the foot, *(see Fig. 36)*. Bunions are almost an epidemic amongst Western women and some studies report that nine out of ten bunion sufferers, are women. The degree of protrusion may vary from person to person - from a small swelling to a severe distortion of the foot. Obviously, the degree of distortion will affect the ability to walk, will cause discomfort and will often mean using special shoe inserts, etc.

As the base of the toe bone pushes outwards, so the big toe itself is often twisted inwards and may squash the second toe out of alignment, which in some cases then overlaps the third toe. Other toes can also be affected by the bunion due to pressure from the big toe pushing inward. Corns and/or other irritations, caused by the overlap of the first and second toes, can also occur. The skin and deeper tissues around the bunion may also be red, swollen, inflamed and callused. Toenails may begin to grow into the sides of the nail bed and the smaller toes can become bent (hammer toes).

Pain from a bunion can be mild, moderate or severe. Bunions are a progressive disease and will, according to most medical opinion, become worse, meaning that once the deformity begins, it will continue to produce greater deformity.

ORIGIN OF THE WORD
The medical name for a bunion is Hallux (Great Toe) Abducto Valgus or (HAV). The word bunion is first found in Latin where it translates as *bunio* meaning enlargement. Later it is found in French where it means lumps or swelling. In the old Anglicized version, it translates as lumps on head. This is interesting in light of the fact that the bunion is found on the toe known in medical circles as the great toe and is related in the study of the feet to the fifth/six/seventh chakras, which physically represent the head and neck. This cannot be coincidental. Clearly the ancient medicine people, who coined the term, must, at some level,

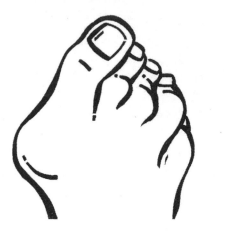

Fig. 36
Bunions

have been aware of the relationship of the big toe to the head.

Bunions can also occur on the outside of the foot along the little toe, where they are called a bunionette or tailor's bunion.

FURTHER EXAMINATION OF PHYSICAL CAUSES

Shoes: In medical circles, tight-fitting shoes especially high heel and narrow-toed shoes, is the generally accepted reason why women are seen to suffer more from bunions than men. Bunions are reported to be more prevalent in people who wear shoes than in people who predominately go barefoot. (This may also be seen as having more to do with the psyche of tribal people than their lack of footwear.)

Let's examine the first cause a bit further. Wearing stilettos does not explain why men who don't wear this type of footwear get bunions. It also offers no explanation as to why some women who wear these shoes don't get bunions. Likewise, many women who have never worn stilettos do get bunions. Shoes do not explain why some people only get the bunion on one foot, or why it is more pronounced on one foot than the other. If wearing shoes were the cause, would it not be logical for the bunions on both feet to be the same? In summary: while it can undoubtedly be a *cause,* wearing high-heeled shoes does not necessarily *result* in bunions – other factors must come into play.

Genetic: A bunion is not something you are born with; rather it develops later in life. It is a deviation from the normal growth of the foot and there are no obvious indications at birth for its possible development. Whereas flatfeet are genetic, as the formation of the foot at birth indicates a predisposition to this problem.

Bunions, as a result of flat feet, could then be said to result as a secondary aspect of genetically inherited flat feet. Although bunions tend to run in families, the foot type is passed down - not the bunion. This could be attributed to a mindset that is passed on from one generation to the next and that may be a relevant emotional trigger.

SPONTANEOUS DEVELOPMENT OF BUNIONS AS A RESULT OF INJURY.

There are numerous instances of bunions developing spontaneously i.e. not through shoes or from flat feet. One instance was that of a 35-year old woman who, while moving furniture, dropped a couch on the base of her big toe, which subsequently developed into a bunion. This could be easily be explained by the weight of the couch forcing the bone outwards, except for the fact that a week later, a bunion developed on the unharmed foot.

Another case that I was witnessed, was that of a woman who stumbled and injured her right foot, which later developed a bunion. A few months later, the left foot also developed a bunion. This type of sympathetic occurrence seems fairly common.

Other risk factors for the development of bunions include congenital abnormal formation of the bones of the foot, nerve conditions that affect the foot, rheumatoid arthritis, abnormality in foot function, injury to the foot and certain occupations that place undue stress on the feet (e.g. ballet dancers and nurses for instance, often develop the condition).

FLAT FEET

With people who have flat feet, the unsupported arch can collapse, shifting the weight of the body unevenly onto the foot, which in some cases causes the bone of the big toe to splay outwards. However, not all people with flat feet develop bunions; in most cases the collapsed arch comes more as a result of the bunion rather than the cause of it.

EMOTIONAL CAUSES

If we examine people who have developed bunions as a result of flat feet, we find an interesting emotional progression. We know that flat feet are a result of not feeling supported or having one's support system collapse. As a child, if one felt unsupported emotionally or financially, it would be hard as an adult, to be a supportive parent. So it makes sense that this affliction could be passed from on generation to another, emotionally and physically.

If a child has not experienced support, nurturing and bonding with its mother, he or she will not feel supported by the universe in later life. Not feeling supported is an issue of trust, i.e. you do not trust the universe to support you. Flat-footed people could be said to have issues relating to trust (first chakra), which relates to feeling ungrounded or not rooted. Lacking trust and grounding results in feeling insecure. We may feel as if we are always getting *swept off our feet* as we struggle to feel safe in a world we do not trust. We feel disconnected from our physical selves and question our right to exist. Chances are that if our mother did not bond with us, she did not feel supported in her role as mother and so, rather than giving us the nurturance and care we needed, she kept from us that which she had not received. She may then have replaced love with discipline and rigid boundaries, or invaded our personal space.

DISCIPLINE AND BUNIONS

"Spare the rod and spoil the child" was a very popular saying at the first part of the 20th century. Our fathers in the past have also been charged with over-disciplining their children or being angry and absent in today's vernacular. This legacy of lack of nurturance was passed from one generation to the next and was exacerbated during the stiff-upper-lip Victorian age, where affection and nurturance was seen as an indulgence not a right.

Why this should have affected more girls than boys, may possibly be due to the fact that boys were commonly the desired sex. Also, there is often a very strong bond between mothers and sons – so boys may be more supported and nurtured as babies than girls. Men in the past were also more able to maintain themselves financially than their female counterparts, who had to rely on their husbands or fathers for financial support.

In this scenario where nurturing is limited, discipline often becomes the prime way of relating to one's offspring. This is a common factor amongst many of the cases I have experienced and all confessed to having been rigidly disciplined by one or both parents, usually the father.

From this lack of support or grounding, comes a deep need to prove to the world that we do have a right to exist and in not feeling secure with who we are and the world around us, we will strive to achieve.

Thus, in order to get approval, we feel we must push ourselves harder and harder in order to meet our parents' expectations. Our constant failure to do so may only push us further to succeed. The withdrawal of approval becomes a way for the parent to manipulate our behaviour and to ensure that they remain the custodians of our power.

It is from this rigidity then that our bunions develop; the heart reflexes push outwards to try to be noticed and to gain the love not received as a child. Because it also touches the fifth chakra, the bunion sufferer may also struggle to express love and emotions to others. The red and swollen area on the skin reveals the anger and emotional pain caused by not feeling nurtured enough. "Look here," the bunion says, "notice me, love me, take care of me." The redness also indicates anger at oneself for not feeling or being good enough and for spending so much time and effort trying to please others. We feel squashed and restricted by not being able to express who we are, so we battle to squash our feet into shoes, which mirror our confined and limited emotions.

Most bunion sufferers also have large calluses over the heart reflex (*see Fig. 37*), which indicates how vulnerable they will feel when it comes to opening their heart to love and emotional expression. One person described the pain from the bunion, as being "like when someone takes a very, very sharp knife or poker and sticks it in the side of your foot," literally like sticking a knife through your heart. The pain reflects the heartfelt distress, which the bunion sufferer may not allow himself or herself to express.

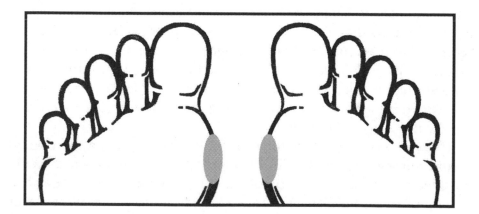

Fig. 37 · Callus on the heart reflex

BUNIONS AND ARTHRITIS

It is common for bunions to progress to arthritis. (Twice as many women as men suffer from arthritis in general, as mentioned previously.) In arthritis, waste toxins in the connective tissue are not released and crystallize which, in feeling terms, translates as a hardening of the emotions. Stiffness results and indicates the arthritic sufferer's own difficulty with change. Similarly, the arthritic sufferer battles to be flexible both in emotions and physical movement.

Sometimes the need to verify one's existence is replaced by the need to excel, resulting not in collapsed arches, but rather raised ones, an indication of perfectionism, which is also the nature of the arthritic sufferer.

This progression from bunions to arthritis, becomes more easily understood when we realize that the arthritic sufferer is manifesting in their feet the physical rigidity that was apparent emotionally in their childhood, i.e. becoming as rigid as our upbringing. In a sense we have come full circle.

CASE STUDIES

Many bunion sufferers seem to be trapped by a difficulty to alter the circumstances of their lives and many suppress their own needs in order to please others, as these example show.

Case one: Sue was a woman that I worked with, who was an extremely good example of this. She was tall and attractive, with gorgeous jet-black hair. Yet in spite of her beauty, her whole demeanour lacked confidence. She sat down nervously on the edge of the chair, and it was hard to believe that she was most at ease in front of an audience. (I recalled that well-known actor, Gerald Depardieu, stuttered off screen.) I concluded then that on stage, she was able to adopt a self-confident persona and in doing so shed her own inhibitions. From what she told me of her past, she was clearly a very talented actress, but since marrying an older man and having three children, she had had to forsake this aspect of her life.

This was hard for her, as the drudgery of carpooling, a tight budget and housework, was no substitution for the stimulation of being on-stage. As the children grew older, she joined a local acting group staging small productions; but this was a far cry from the stage career of her youth. In spite of this, however, she enjoyed the thrill of appearing behind the footlights and all seemed to be well until her husband began to object to her late nights, a part and parcel of being in these productions.

Her husband, who was a very insecure and controlling man, had been very threatened by her success and belittled her achievements to the point of refusing to come and see her on stage. As time went on he became more and more resentful of the happiness that seemed to exclude him and ordered her to stop acting. Obviously resentful of his curtailment to the first real happiness she had found in years, the decision put a strain on the marriage.

It was at this time that she tripped and fell. (Symbolically this mirrored her difficulty in moving forward.) Shortly after this, a bunion developed on her right foot and later on her left foot.

In chatting to her, we spoke about confronting her husband and telling him how unhappy his decision had made her. She was reluctant to do this firstly, because he had a violent temper and she was afraid of his reaction and secondly, because she had come to doubt her ability to act. What if she did rebel against him only to find she was rejected by the acting world? The humiliation would be huge. Rather, she chose to live her life unfulfilled and resentful of his actions.

She also had netlike lines on the second and third chakras – (an indication that she felt trapped). When I asked her if she could relate to this, she agreed and yet she did not know how to free herself. She blamed others for her entrapment and consequently did not feel empowered to move. Any suggestion I made to the contrary was met with resistance (i.e. fear). She felt she had to martyr her needs (in this case her acting career) for the sake of maintaining her marriage, whereas the truth lay more in her own fear of making a change and setting new boundaries in the relationship.

This was a very miserable situation for the whole family as when a mother is unfulfilled and unhappy in her life, it affects all members of the family. I wondered if the restrictions this man had placed on his wife, were worth the disharmony that permeated the home. If he had had the courage to give her the freedom to find herself (even at the risk of losing her) the possible reward of a happy, fulfilled relationship would surely have been worth it.

Case two: I was told a story of a young woman who grew up in the early 1900s in Cape Town, South Africa who was a brilliant and very gifted singer. In spite of her achievements at University in the music academy, her father refused to allow her to take up the bursary offered to her to study further overseas with one of the top teachers. Singing, in his opinion, was no job for a woman.

Disillusioned, she married the first man who came along, a farmer who took her away from the little teaching she was receiving, to his farm in the semi-desert, desolate Karoo. She proved a dutiful wife, producing three children, before contracting tuberculosis.

Tuberculosis is a disease of the lungs and because of the difficulty it causes in breathing, it represents an inability to breathe freely or to take in life fully. With TB patients often get pneumonia, which indicates a tiredness for life and desperation with the situation they find themselves in. Together with the TB, pneumonia causes internal bleeding and this blood is coughed up. Blood makes up a large part of our bodies and is the symbol of our life force. Through its composition, our individuality is expressed. When we cough it up, we expel our life force. Instead of breathing out stale air we cough up our very essence. TB also has to do with revenge, which this unfortunate woman understandably wanted to wreak on her father and husband. She was sent away to recover, which removed her from her children and husband. (Given the combination of revenge, a draining of life force and lack of freedom, it's understandable why TB raged with such fury in South Africa during the years of apartheid.)

After a lengthy recovery, she returned to the farm, but later was encouraged by a friend to attend an audition in the city, adjudicated by a famous international teacher. The very dour teacher told the woman that she would tell her straight out if felt she had talent.

Upon hearing her voice, the teacher started to cry and identified her as the most talented singer she had encountered. She was once again offered the opportunity to train in Europe and this time it was her husband who refused to let her go. Trapped in the unsophisticated confines of a small town whose inhabitants were unable to appreciate her talent, she gave up any hope of singing professionally. In never receiving the approval of an audience and living with a husband who never appreciated or wanted to appreciate the extent of her ability, the love and approval she craved eluded her.

Throughout her life she suffered from severe bunions, which made walking very painful. I suspect if I had been able to examine her feet there would have been a huge callus across the heart area too. Once again the theme of restriction and sublimating one's desires to please others reappears in this story. She was never able to find the means to stand up against the dominant male figures in her life in order to explore her undoubted talent. Instead she died unknown, bitter and unfulfilled.

Case three: Sylvia was the founder of a large retail chain. She was short, verging on tubby, with hunched shoulders - not exactly the image of a highly successful businesswoman. She also had large bunions on both feet. She responded passionately when asked about her need to please others to the point of sublimating her own desires.

This unhappy woman was not sacrificing her talent, but she had created a situation where, although successful, she felt powerless to change. She was as trapped by her success, as the other women were by their failure to achieve success.

This need to do things correctly and to please her customers, had created a sure fire success and the company had grown to the point where her husband's income was far below her profit. This caused a tension in the marriage as, already verging on abusive, his ego battled to deal with his wife's success. In business she was a success, but at home her husband never stopped reminding her how she failed in so many ways. This drove her even harder to achieve better results and consequently made her feel trapped in her career and constantly exhausted from the stress and strain. Added to that was the guilt she felt at having to ignore many of her children's needs at the expense of being successful.

New stores opened, staff constantly came and went, stocks had to be sourced and ordered, shipments then had to be delivered as the business grew and grew. Yet in time she felt even more trapped and a slave to the needs of the company and its employees. She also felt trapped in a loveless marriage. Although money was not an issue and she freely acknowledged that love did not exist in her marriage, she could not see her way clear to breaking free. She had created a dark hole for herself and could not climb out.

Her red bunions glowed with the anger she felt towards her husband and ached with the pain of an unfulfilled relationship and even while speaking about him during the session, they glowed ever redder. However, she was not prepared to take any real steps to change the situation, fearing the possible consequences. I saw her a year or so later, still looking as stressed, still in far too much of a rush to actually enjoy any of her successes and, from what she told me in the brief time I had with her, the marital situation had worsened. Still she refused to budge from the world she had created.

I am always deeply saddened by situations like this, as I have also seen the other side of the coin when people do realize they have climbed to the top of a long ladder only to discover they chose the wrong ladder. By then it's often too late to scramble down and climb up the other one.

THE BUNION CYCLE

While no one individual responds exactly like another there is a general pattern to bunions, some or all of which may apply to you if you suffer from them:

- In childhood, our thoughts, feelings and desires are restricted and limited by the rigidity of others.
- This can lead to a striving to achieve the thoughts, feelings and desires of others.
- This in turn becomes a desire to be perfect/perfectionism.
- Perfectionism can lead to restricted self-expression, lack of self-worth and insecurity.
- Then there can be a fear of starting something in case it might fail, or else we push ourselves very hard to achieve.
- This can result in anger and resentment when approval is not forthcoming.
- It can also cause feelings of being trapped – our insecurity binds us to situations and unexpressed feelings.
- Then this leads to stuckness, which causes rigidity within ourselves, even as we cry out for love.

BUNIONS WITH NO FOOT ARCH
ISSUES OR ARTHRITIS

Many people who have bunions have neither arch (support issues) nor arthritis (needing love/critical of self and others). However, I suspect that almost all who suffer from bunions have had a strict or rigid upbringing and most often it is the father figure who rules with a rod of iron. In a world of withheld emotions and/or conditional love, the bunion sufferer reaches out for love and approval, and where there is a strong disciplinarian figure, the person with bunions is also afraid to *take a stand* or *stand on their own two feet* and say what they think or feel for fear of derision from the strict parental figure. Therefore, they try to meet the needs of their parents at the expense of their own.

Bunion sufferers seem at times stifled by troubled emotions that they struggle to express and so cannot move on from them. These people so wanted to excel that it hurt and angered them when they failed to achieve the high standards they set for themselves.

(IT'S) TRYING TO BE PERFECT

Because of this desire for perfection, many bunion sufferers are drawn to sports or activities that require intense self-discipline. Those dedicated to the martial arts, ballet dancing and yoga are all disciplines where I found not only a predominance of bunions, but also a determination to follow careers involving much self-sacrifice and long hard hours.

In America where women are taught to achieve, bunions are extremely common. Women often work long hours, sacrificing themselves by not having kids, etc., all in the name of achievement and in an attempt to be seen as equal to men. This need may become so consuming and keep them so occupied, that they may lose touch with their emotions. Being unaware of how they feel, they are unable to align their personality to their soul. This, combined with the strong desire to live up to the expectations of others, indicates that in many cases they will not be able to connect with their authentic selves. Being unable to do so, they remain frustrated and unfulfilled. The need to excel, be appreciated and noticed manifests in the bunion, which pushes itself out to gain recognition but may, in its enlarged state, contain much emotional garbage which the sufferer finds hard to express, or even connect with.

The inability of the toe to move to its original position indicates that inflexibility is an issue. The big toe (relating to thoughts) may indicate trouble either in making decisions or changing existing ideas. We may be held captive to others or our own decisions or may struggle to make our thoughts manifest.

Chris Stormer, author and reflexologist, describes bunion sufferers as people where *"Inflexibility gives the impression of bigotry."*[2] Broken down, the word bigotry relates not only to the narrowness of ideas, but also to the need for perfectionism: *Big- o(n)- try!* which is a fair summation of bunion suffererers.

OTHER INTERESTING COMMON FEATURES

Most people with bunions have thick calluses over the heart and often over the little toe, indicating a vulnerability and a need to protect oneself in issues of the heart and, if on the small toe, from their family, which makes sense if loving was replaced with discipline in childhood. Where all the toes splay off to the side, they may have experienced all own their own thoughts, expression and ideas having been pushed aside.

Yellow feet are also common, indicating just how fed up their owners are with having to please others and suppress their own emotional and physical needs.

Several people have have told me that when they have had conflict with their partners, their bunions have flared up and become more red and painful.

The desire to please others often manifests in a need to serve others. So, bunion sufferers are often very caring people or drawn to fields involved in the inspiring others. Teaching is a popular interest or career, not necessarily in a school per se, but more often in areas to assist in the enlightenment of others, for instance, or in the arts, such as ballet, drama, writing, art, martial arts, etc. Perhaps this is because teaching combines discipline with assisting others, and also gives them the positive reinforcement they need from their pupils. Often they are the people in the family who give the nurturance and care for everyone else. Through their service to others, they may martyr themselves or *push themselves hard*, i.e. suffer or repress their own needs in order to assist others.

HEALING

Traditional treatments: non-invasive methods vary from simply wearing protective pads, altering the type of shoes you wear, inserting good arch supports or having shoes professionally-stretched to surgery.

Over 130 operations for bunions have been described. Generally, surgery would involve realigning the bone, ligaments and tendons so that the big toe can revert to its original position. A simple Bunionectomy can be done if the condition is mild and it is a relatively minor procedure. The Keller procedure is a bit more complicated and involves the removal of part of the joint of the big toe, as well as tightening the ligaments. It can be problematic, as the toe bone is shortened and part of the toe which now has no bone, can become floppy. (I saw this happen to one of my clients where the bone of the squashed toe had been removed.) Not only is this procedure cosmetically unsightly for the reasons given but the deformity may also reoccur.

An Osteotomy involves cutting the bones and re-directing them in a straighter position. This altered bone is then held together with pins, screws or in a cast for 6-8 weeks. This method is the best aesthetically, but involves crutches and a longer recuperation time, as well as greater expense. The bone also does not always heal correctly and further surgery is required in some instances.

In soft tissue procedures, the surgeon tightens ligaments and transfers muscles in order to correct the deformity, so the toe is pulled in the opposite direction. This may be done in addition to one of the above procedures or as a procedure on its own. Disadvantages include the toe pulling too far in the opposite direction and thereby creating equal problems and necessitating further surgery.

EMOTIONAL HEALING

Most of the clients I have seen with bunions have with filled me with a deep sense of loss for what might have been in their lives. If they had been able to let go of the need to gain others' approval or not feel quite so obliged to assist others at their own expense, they might have freed themselves up to achieve their own ambitions. So much of their lives seemed to have been a constant, hard struggle, where they often felt alone and incapable of changing their situations.

To heal emotionally, they need to acknowledge their repressed feelings and approve of themselves, rather than wait for the unforthcoming approval of others; in addition, they need to let go of the need to be perfect. To be is all they need to be.

Burning Feet

KEY ISSUES
A situation that we have smouldered over. A history of unexpressed anger. Inability to let go of anger and move forward.

PHYSICAL CAUSES
Burning feet occur when your feet feel as if they are permanently positioned next to a very warm heater. It is most commonly found in people over 50 years of age. Medically speaking, there are many different causes. Diabetics are the most common sufferers, while alcoholics are also susceptible. However, there are many other causes for this sensation, such as thyroid dysfunction, gastric restriction in obese people, excessively sweaty feet, nerve entrapment syndrome (such as tarsal tunnel syndrome) or a pinched nerve between the third and fourth toes.

EMOTIONAL CAUSES
When we experience the sensation of our feet burning, it is an emotional indication that we are angry or incensed about a situation, which quite possibly has been *smouldering* for years.

In the case of *diabetes*, we may be fuming over what we perceive as a lack of sweetness in our lives or the inability to control the people around us. On a physical level, diabetics cannot absorb sugar in food, which is mirrored emotionally by the difficulty they have accepting love, or the sweetness in life, either a lack of love, or from being smothered with love. There is also a link with diabetes and *obesity*, which makes sense when one considers that over-eating is a way we compensate for a lack of love in our lives. As we feel our feet burn, we are burning with both the need for love and the anger at it not being given.

In the case of *alcoholics*, we are infuriated and disillusioned with how our lives have panned out, and feel inadequate or unworthy of being loved; however, not receiving it enrages us and our feet *feel the heat*.

Louise Hay, author of *Heal Your Body*, writes that the *thyroid* is related to humiliation.[2] When we suffer from thyroid dysfunction and our feet feel as if they are burning, we may be extremely angry at whoever has humiliated us, and being in the area of the throat, perhaps also at ourselves for not standing up to them.

Tarsal Tunnel Syndrome is similar to Carpal Tunnel Syndrome (which affects the wrist.) The tibial nerve becomes trapped in the Tarsal Tunnel of the ankle. Common causes for entrapment include an enlarged adjacent muscle, a cyst, flat feet, rheumatoid arthritis, a fracture or diabetes. It usually worsens as the day progresses. Nerves are the body's communicators: if we put our hand on a hot plate it is the nerves that send the message to the brain, "Hey, lift the hand up." When a nerve is trapped, it symbolizes a block in communication, or an area in our lives where we feel trapped. The burning feet mirror the frustration and anger we feel at this situation. The ankles support our bodies so we may feel trapped in some way in areas having to do with support and with the ability to move freely, and are angry consequently.

In the case of the cause being a *pinched nerve* between the third and fourth toes, we know from the chakras in Chapter Two, that these toes relate to issues to do with our relationship to ourselves and our one-on-one relationships. With the nerve being pinched here, we clearly are experiencing a block in communicating, or expressing our ideas, or beliefs, which may be causing pain and anger towards others and ourselves.

CASE STUDY

An elderly woman, Lillian, complained of a burning sensation under her feet in the heart chakra area which she had experienced for a number of years. (*see Fig. 38*)

She had visited doctors, podiatrists and a number of other specialists in the hope of curing this irritating condition. Nothing had resulted in a permanent cure, and it was on the recommendation of her daughter

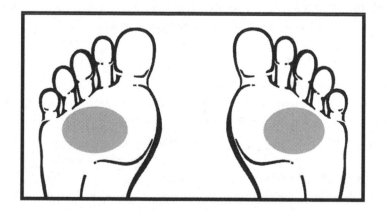

Fig. 38 · Burning areas on the heart

that we met. She was not averse to alternative healing, although she was skeptical that it would be beneficial; however, she did agree to let me examine her feet. She had been widowed for several years following a long and relatively happy marriage. In conversation with her it became apparent that she had never discovered the "I am," within herself. She had played roles, such as "I am a housewife"; "I am Fred's wife; or "I am a mother," but acknowledged that these were simply roles beneath which she had never had the time or space to discover who she really was.

For years she had sublimated her will to the needs of her husband and children. Whatever they wanted came first and what she wanted was always suppressed. Now in her late sixties, she finally had the space and time to find herself, but had no idea where and what to look for. She could not blame her offspring or husband now, but had to look inside herself for the solution. She became angry at her own fears and lack of ability to act courageously, not to mention all the years she perceived she had wasted. She was also angry with herself feeling that in many ways she had held her husband back from exploring new projects and ideas. All the years of smouldering over her unexpressed anger, both at herself and her unfulfilled life, had caused the burning sensation in her feet, in the heart chakra, just below the third toe. She longed to love herself, yet she did not know who she really was, so there wasn't anyone really to love.

Rather than forgive and release issues from the past, she held onto her history which burnt her up. She was able to see the pattern that she had created and to release some of the anger. In doing so, I felt sure that the sensation would lesson and that she would free herself up energetically to fully embrace the remaining years.

PHYSICAL HEALING

The pain and burning sensation can usually be temporarily relieved by rest, bathing feet in cool water, elevation, wearing cotton socks, or massage. Arch supports, wider shoes, steroid injections may help and, in extreme cases, surgery may be required.

EMOTIONAL HEALING

Examine what issues may be making you fume. Having identified the issue, work at ways to release this anger – without taking a mallet to the perceived perpetrator! This may require working with issues of self-esteem in order to reach the point where one can, calmly and straight-forwardly, address the issue(s) that have and still do anger you. E.g. "What you are doing is not acceptable to me, because I find it x, y and z; could you please stop doing it? Thanks." Anger frequently masks our fear and hurt and, to fully release the burning sensation/anger, we may need to resolve these emotions, perhaps through accepting responsibility for what has happened, and then forgiving both ourselves and who-ever else may be involved.

Realise that your anger is not you. It is simply an energetic pattern that you have identified with. Your thoughts and emotions are not who you are. Learn to acknowledge your anger, allow yourself to feel it without judgement. Then be aware that once you have done this it will dissipate.

Chilblains

KEY ISSUES

Fear of intimacy or contact. Feeling vulnerable and exposed. Numbed by experiences. Issues needing to be voiced, often anger. Fear of conflict.

PHYSICAL CAUSES

Chilblains are red, sore and often itchy swellings that can appear on the fingers, toes and, less commonly, on the nose or ears. In severe cases the skin can actually burst and a secondary infection can set in. Chilblains are caused by poor circulation to these extremities (often from a damaged blood vessel due to exposure to cold). Dampness can compound the problem and the skin is more likely to burst if wet. Tight fitting shoes can also cut off the circulation to the toes, resulting in chilblains. Principally though, poor circulation is the problem.

EMOTIONAL CAUSES

Taking the first issue into account, namely the redness, indicates some anger at situations or events that are causing us pain. The itchiness is an indication of something that needs to surface or that is *itching for attention*. Like an insect bite, something is bugging us. We are tempted to scratch to relieve the pressure and itchiness; however no amount of scratching seems to help. This frustration shows us that we are angry with someone or something yet feel unable either to release the issue or confront it. Should the skin burst, the watery ooze that emerges is the watery tears that have burst our seams. Sadness is often masked by anger and may be behind the frustration that we are afraid of voicing. Interestingly, outside damp (outside emotional issues) leads to this internal eruption.

The cold that we feel externally indicates how numbed our emotions have become. We are frozen by our fear of voicing our anguish, which causes this build-up or swelling. We have developed *cold feet*, indicating our fear of moving ahead. Obviously seeing which toes are affected will determine what this pain and conflict relates to.

Poor circulation reveals that we want to withdraw from life. We feel weak and unable to stand up for ourselves and lack vitality. We renounce our power and are unable to circulate lovingly in our lives.

Blood circulates in our bodies giving us life. Being water, the female element, it symbolises love and emotion. Poor circulation means we do not want to enter into this process. We fear not only living fully, but also emotional involvement and love or intimacy. Like tortoises, we pull in our heads, legs and tails as a way to protect ourselves from feeling vulnerable. We cannot reach out for love, for we fear it and freeze ourselves emotionally. Doing so causes us frustration and pain.

CASE STUDY

A young girl I met, who was approximately eight or nine, had large chilblains on both her small toes. She was not a client for this was some years ago, but rather she was someone whom I met in the course of my daily life. I was reminded of her and her chilblains whilst writing this section and decided to include the pieces of her story that I remembered, because the incidents in her life, I felt, related to her chilblains which she had almost constantly, in spite of living in South Africa where temperatures are relatively warm.

She was a quiet child as I recall, withdrawn, with brooding blue eyes and a great love of animals. She was the youngest of four children. There was sadness in this child that I could not explain, given her apparently stable, middle-class home. Later I learned that at the time I met her and when she had chilblains, this child was being sexually abused by a family member. Now this is not to say that all people with chilblains are being sexually abused, but rather that this was an extreme case of someone who for obvious reasons felt the need to withdraw from the painful world around them.

No wonder she feared contact and intimacy, when her youthful experience of it had been one of fear, guilt and manipulation. So great was her shock at the experiences, that she had for many years erased them from her conscious recollection. She had numbed herself to not only those experiences, but all others. Powerless to voice her anger at the violation of her body, her toes swelled with unresolved emotions. The perpetrator was much older and a respected family member, whom she felt powerless to confront. No doubt the conflict between wanting to please this person yet also feeling guilty for what she knew was wrong created confusion in her young mind. She loved this person, yet they abused that love and she felt powerless to react. She also recounted that she had feared no-one would believe her if she exposed him and her fear was then of being ostracized from the family, who would not take kindly to her revelations. She could not then voice her anger. Rather she withdrew into the world of animals, which she could trust and love, without fear of being abused.

The chilblains were mostly on the baby toes, indicating that the issues lay within the family and her insecurity within her relationships there. Occasionally they did appear on her fourth toes, as a sign of how much toxic emotion she had towards the perpetrator. Years later, through therapy, she confronted her demons and released many of the painful experiences of her childhood. Gradually she started to enter fully into life, and tentatively explore more intimate relationships. The chilblains did not return even when she moved to the colder climate of England.

HEALING

What emotions are you feeling numbed to? Who or what makes you feel vulnerable? Has someone invaded your boundaries and made you want to withdraw? What stops you from expressing how you feel? When we become frozen with fear, we cannot move and must live in the situation constantly. Only by melting our frozen water with fire/anger can we hope to free ourselves from the situation. Often the situations we confront are far less threatening than when we withdraw from them.

Corns and Calluses

KEY ISSUES

Hardening of self to protect one's vulnerability. Shutting off. Not wanting to see, hear, speak, feel, etc.

PHYSICAL CAUSES

Corns and calluses are thickenings of the surface layer of skin caused by pressure and friction on the skin of your foot. Usually they can be seen easily and may have a tender spot in the middle, surrounded by yellowish dead skin.

They may occur when bones of the foot press against the shoe or when two foot bones press together. Together with calluses, they are the feet's most common problem. Corns usually are found where the bone is prominent and presses the skin against the shoe, ground, or other bones, whereas calluses usually appear on the sides or underneath the foot. Hard corns are usually located on the top of the toe or on the side of the small toe. Soft corns resemble open sores and develop between the toes as they rub against each other. They both involve a thickening (hyperkeratosis) of the outer layer of the skin, but whereas corns tend to be smaller and circular in size, calluses can be quite large. As corns become thick, the tissue under the corn becomes increasingly irritated. A core may develop where the corn is thickest. As corns become inflamed, there is pain and sometimes swelling and redness, particularly at the core. Treatment involves relieving the pressure on the skin, usually by modifying the shoe. Pads to relieve the bony pressure are helpful, if positioned carefully. On occasion, surgery is necessary to remove a bony prominence that causes the corn or callus.

Like bunions, corns occur more in women than in men. Their occurrence has been attributed to tight-fitting shoes; shoes that are too large and where the foot slides around; socks that chafe; deformed, hammer or skew toes; a seam inside a shoe that causes friction; and downhill walking. Obviously removing or moderating these causes may help, although it has been my experience that while alleviating the pain, the corn is seldom removed. Corn-removing solutions should be used with extreme care due to the acid they contain and, according to information I have, should not be used by diabetics and those with poor circulation, all of whom should seek professional help because of the serious consequences of infection.

COMPLICATIONS THAT CAN RESULT FROM CORNS

Sometimes a fluid-filled sac called bursitis can develop underneath the corn; infection and ulcers (some extending down to the bone) can also develop. This makes walking painful and the restraint of movement mirrors emotionally the anger at not being able to move freely.

SELF-TREATMENT

This could involve soaking your feet regularly, using a pumice stone to reduce the size of the corn or callus, wearing a foam pad over the corn for protection and placing lamb's wool between the toes to act as a cushion. (If you are a diabetic, have diminished circulation, or other sensations, you need to consult a medical practitioner.)

ORIGIN OF WORD

Corn means a small seed or grain, as well as to wear away. Because of its resemblance to a piece of corn, it was later used to describe the hard yellow skin on the foot as 'corn on the foot.' A callus comes from the Latin *callosus*, meaning thick-skinned or hard-skinned, from where its figurative sense as in 'unfeeling' appeared. Note that although the spelling of the physical "callus" is different from the feeling "callous," they both have the same origins.

COLOURS OF CALLUSES AND CORNS

If the callus is yellow it indicates that we are really pissed-off with the situation. More often than not corns are yellow, indicating underlying frustration and feeling disgruntled. When the callus appears to be white, this could indicate complete exhaustion – literally, feeling drained (of colour). If the corn is red it would reflect anger.

EMOTIONAL CAUSES

Both corns and calluses involve a thickening of the skin and, as the terms *callous* and *thick-skinned* implies, they are to do with insensitivity. We become this way either because of our emotional need to protect ourselves from others, where we have been hurt or threatened (desensitizing us where we feel most vulnerable) or in areas where we have become shut off or hardened to our *own* feelings. Corns, because they are found primarily on the toes (toes have to do with ideas and thinking,) indicate where we have become hardened to our thoughts; whereas a callus, on the heart area, indicates where we have become hardened to our feelings. Sometimes a sac of fluid builds up under the callus, indicating bottled-up emotions. Exactly where the corns or calluses appear, will give us a better idea as to what specific areas are involved. Here is a description of the most common areas where corns and calluses are found.

CORNS ON SPECIFIC TOES

Corns most commonly appear on the toes, which represent the fifth, sixth and seventh chakras. From Chapter Two, we know that the main toe-related issues in these chakras involve self-expression, insight or intuition, and our thoughts. Developing a thick skin in these areas could mean that we wish to shield ourselves from our own thoughts, or from others who may belittle or deride them.

When corns are found on the toe pad, we may not want to be aware of our inner voice and consequently block it off. We do not want to see what is really happening. Should the corns appear on the sides of the toes (where the ear reflexes are found) we do not want to hear the truth, or we shut ourselves off from that which we find distasteful. Lower down on the neck of the toe, would mean we resist expressing our ideas or thoughts. Or that we defend them against the perceived attack of others.

The toe on which the corn appears is important in relation to what particular aspects of thoughts or ideas are requiring defense or cocooning. Briefly, the *small toe*, or first toe, has to do with thoughts about family, or work situations. This toe is a very common place for a corn, quite simply because it is very often our families who attack our beliefs, ideas or thinking. When our our families or colleagues constantly belittle our thoughts, the only way we can cope is to construct a defensive wall, so we can't hear them and also so we don't have to hear our own voice, which is probably telling us to move on. We have to become hardened to their ridicule or lack of approval.

When the corn falls on the *second toe*, our defensiveness would become more personal, involving a spouse, friend, sibling, particular colleague, etc. We may not want to deal with thoughts about a particular person, or we may be defending ourselves against their attack on our thoughts. The foot on which the corn appears could also relate to whether the person involved was male (right foot) or female (left foot) or what aspects of our own inner male/female are involved.

On the *third toe*, the focus would shift more to our relationship towards our self-esteem and ourselves. We may be sabotaging our own ideas by telling ourselves we lack the skill and/or talent to follow up on our thoughts, or we may feel the lack of acceptance of our ideas from others, is a personal slight to ourselves. The fourth toe has to do with matters of the heart and how we give and receive love, both to others and ourselves. Corns here could mean we are defending our thoughts about love or have built up a wall to protect ourselves from feeling pain about past hurts. The big toe representing the top three chakras, as listed above, has already been covered.

CORNS WITH ULCERS

The word ulcer, according to the *Oxford Dictionary*, means a *corroding or corrupting influence*. When ulcers form on a corn on the toes, they imply that our thoughts or our beliefs are eating us up, or that thoughts of painful experiences are corroding us. Often they appear on the softer corns between the toes, where we find the ear reflexes. This barrier and its corrosion would imply that we don't want hear the thoughts that are eating us up.

CALLUSES ON THE HEEL OF THE FOOT

Commonly calluses appear on or around the heel of the foot, which is associated with the first chakra. So, issues to examine would be those of family/corporation/ groups of people that we perceive may be stopping us moving ahead. Often people who are very stuck will manifest an extra bit of heel at the back of the foot, which mirrors their immobility. It is as if they struggle to break away from the family or groups of people they are connected with, to discover their own path. (This could vary from a tribal way of living in the sense of indigenous people, to being associated with a particular type of career or profession whose values you have allowed yourself to be governed by.)

Perhaps we are *digging our heels in* and refusing to shift because we are afraid of what the future holds. We do not *trust the ground we step on* to provide for our needs and so we resist the call to change. We are afraid to find our own way ahead as it would mean leaving the security of the known, or the group we belong to.

If the callus has become cracked on the heel, the issue is literally *cracking us up*, making it painful to progress. Perhaps we have security issues that have developed cracks and are making us feel insecure.

CASE STUDY

Case one: One client had very large corns on the tops of his third and fourth toes, requiring the wearing of shoe pads. This man was brilliant, but was continually being put down by his wife, to the point that they barely communicated. When they did, it usually involved him being told that whatever his plans (thoughts) may have been, they were unacceptable to her. Now, obviously there were many others aspects leading up to this inharmonious relationship, but his corns indicated that he had built up a thick defense to her onslaught. And, as his toes curled backwards, they also showed just how hammered down this man was.

Case two: Imagine living alone with your daughter for most of your life, after having suffered a heart-wrenching breakup (the line across her heart chakra was testimony to this) in your early twenties, with a new baby and no support. This was the situation with Jane, a short woman in her fifties. She came to see me on the advice of her daughter who had also been a client of mine. As she was in the accounting field, she was by nature a practical person and had not experienced much in the way of alternate healing modalities.

Without going into all the details about her feet, she did display a characteristic which was relevant to the very large corn on her right foot. Her arches were especially flat, almost to the point of connecting to the ground. She admitted to feeling unsupported and at times she reached out for support, but had not received it. This was a theme that played itself out in all aspects of her life and was reflected in her foot characteristics.

However, Jane was a great giver and being single with a relatively good income, was constantly required to assist her large family of brothers and sisters (five in all) and, in later years their children. When someone required a lift, Aunty Jane was there; if money was required for school fees, Aunty Jane was top of the list. Because of her reclusive single life, she was a great bet for babysitting, and when it came to family functions Aunty Jane was there to cater for everybody. Now retired, she was tired of being so busy helping everyone, and was resenting the fact that when she had needed help, no-one was around.

I asked about her feelings towards herself when not playing these roles of mother, cook, financial provider, babysitter etc. and her words were, "I am nothing." Through this she could see that she had taken on these roles to be anything that would mask her feelings of inadequacy. Having created the situation, now she had no way to withdraw from these roles in order to find herself. It is interesting that Jane was fifty. Our lives work in seven year cycles, which meant that Jane was just embarking on a new cycle, which clearly had to do with finding her true self.

Jane had a huge corn on the small toe of her right foot (family issues) and a smaller one on the left foot represented the barrier she had to create between herself and her family in order to protect herself. (Her adrenal gland on the left foot was sunken, indicating she was exhausted with the situation.) If she had not created this boundary her family would have simply taken over her life completely. And she, in order to feel needed, would most likely have let them do so. This thick skin was her boundary behind which she hid, unable to express to them her anger at feeling 'used.' As this big corn was over the ear reflex, this indicated that she also did not want to really listen to them and their advice about her life. She wanted to *turn a deaf ear* to the family and their ideas as to how how she should live her life. Everyone had an idea as to why she had not found another man (right toe) and how she should have behaved towards the only real love of her life. This was painful to hear, and so she shut them out, by becoming thickskinned to their advice. Also by not feeding her the approval she needed, the family made sure that she tried even harder to be what they required, making her feel guilty when she did not comply.

No wonder this poor woman developed corns! After a time she came to see that her major responsibility now lay in nurturing herself - in filling her own empty cup. Creativity is a wonderful way to do this. She expressed an interest in Origami, which she said she never had time to explore. Working on a principle in Julia Cameron's book *The Artist's Way,* we spoke about setting up specific appointments (artist's dates) with herself to devote to Origami. Just feeling that it was alright to cut out her family and pursue her own life, was a major step forward for Jane.

The heart is our centre of love (self and others), intimacy and relationship. It's a very common spot for a callus (almost 50% of the people I have seen have a callus of some sort over the heart reflex or

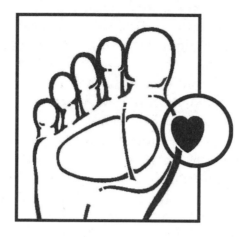

Fig. 39 · Calluses on inner side of foot in the heart area.

heart chakra) and it's not too hard to figure out why! Where does so much of our pain come from? I believe it's the need to love and be loved. Yet this is where we experience so much grief as our hearts often do get broken. So we build these walls around ourselves to shut off our own feelings and not allow others to penetrate our emotional self. It is also common on the actual reflex (as well as over the area in general) to find a deep groove or cut literally indicating a broken heart or being *cut-up*.

Case three: One client who had enormous calluses on both feet, was a young, tall, thickset man called Steven. He was in his early thirties, unmarried, although in a committed relationship. He had trained as an engineer, but had not worked in this field, preferring the excitement of property development and the stock market. He had experienced considerable success in this field (largely because of his streetwise instinct for survival). Drugs, mostly cocaine, had been an issue when he was flying with the jet-set elite, but he had since stopped taking them. This caused him a problem, as he felt isolated from his old companions, who could not deal with his reformed self. Every now and again he would give in and take drugs, only to stop once more. He came to see me because he was interested in what I did, but also because he got anxious from time to time and could not sleep without taking sleeping tablets - in contradiction to the healthy lifestyle he had now adopted. He was keen on sport, in spite of his nonathletic build.

Regardless of his financial success, his past kept following him, bringing up patterns of rejection and later self-criticism, which he then attempted to escape through the drugs. He could not find anything about himself to love.

He was very jumpy and tense when he got onto my table for Reiki and leapt off it the minute I finished working with him. (Most people prefer to relax for a few minutes, enjoying the peace and tranquility.) He was uncomfortable with being touched and so found the process hard. He found it especially hard to switch off his very active mind so he could actually relax. The same behaviour continued for the next two sessions; following the first of which he had shown signs of detoxification, i.e. cold like symptoms, and acute headaches after the next treatment. He did say, however, that he was experiencing greater periods of calmness and needed fewer sleeping tablets, sometimes none at all to get to sleep.

In spite of these improvements, I felt he was frustrated with the process. It was as if there was so much that he wanted to release but still he held back; so I asked him how he would feel if I looked at his feet, and he agreed to let me do so.

As I looked at his feet, I was aware of how clean and scrubbed they were. (I see a fair number of very dirty and rough-looking feet, particularly with young men who lead outdoor lives.) However, this man's feet were meticulously scrubbed and the nails were trimmed evenly and neatly.

He had large calluses on his heart chakra on both feet, with a particular build-up on the heart (see Fig. 39) as well as a dividing line in the heart chakra – this may be a result of the effect of the separation from his parents he had felt when sent away to boarding school. (Note: not everyone who has been sent to boarding school will have this line; it is simply an indication that the move had caused serious emotional pain in this particular individual.) I asked him whether he had experienced much grief or emotional pain in his life. He replied that his parents had divorced after an unhappy marriage, when he was still quite young, whereupon he and his two siblings had been shipped off to a very old-fashioned, rather draconian boarding school, where he became the target of much bullying.

As the eldest boy he was expected to take care of his two younger brothers. He felt ashamed of his sporting inadequacies and different from the other boys. He had little self-esteem and did not love or even like himself. His inadequacies were constantly highlighted both by his peers and his parents. His way of coping was to cut himself off from his feelings, as this helped him overcome his almost constant fear of being attacked. He lived with this anxiety, fearing both the teachers and the boys.

I suggested that this might be the initial source of the anxiety attacks he was currently experiencing. He agreed. Given this history it was no surprise to see why he had shut himself off from his emotions and at the same time made his heart almost impenetrable.

Speaking further, we examined this fight or flight mentality and why in his career, he now constantly put himself into these situations which threatened his security. On the stock market you can win big, but you can also lose all you have, just as in property speculations, you can burn your fingers badly. It was as if he had become addicted to creating scary situations and when he emerged from them unscathed, he achieved a kind of high. Although enjoying playing the stock market, he experienced major panic attacks and feared every possible thing that could go wrong. However, no sooner had he got out of one such situation than he would invest in some other scheme. He was addicted to risk taking. Living in constant fear was something he had learnt as a child and now he was entrenched in an addictive pattern. The reward of surviving gave him an adrenaline rush or high that was ample reward for the fear he had experienced. It was the only way that he was able to experience living in the present, as opposed to dwelling in the guilt of the past or the fear of the future.

His puffy adrenal reflexes confirmed the presence of constant fear. This, together with his very dysfunctional early family background, as well as his high risk personality, pointed to a much wounded first chakra. I pointed out the deep ridges in the area of his first chakra which indicated the difficulties he had and was still experiencing.

I also asked how easily he was able to give and receive love, as his calluses gave me the impression that he was afraid of intimacy. He said he struggled to open up emotionally to his girlfriends and could never share deep intimacy with them. This inability to make himself vulnerable was causing problems in his current relationship and was, no doubt, why his past relationships had ended. I suggested that perhaps this could be linked to a fear of being rejected and, that in order to work through his fear he would have to have faith and trust both himself and others. Love was an issue for him; he said he felt like an explorer in a foreign land, unsure what it was he was looking for and whether he would know it if he found it. When I suggested this may be because he had not experienced it himself as a child, he agreed and became very emotional. For the first time in many years he was able to let go and release some of the grief that had lived behind the thick callused walls he had created.

Later, we spoke of feelings of being abandoned by his parents and the violence he had experienced at school and later from his father at home. We also addressed the issue of safety and affirmed that his desire to reconnect to his body through sport was a very positive thing to do.

Subsequently, while having Reiki, he actually fell asleep on the massage table and did not leap off the bed as before, but remained relaxed for a few minutes. This was very positive and I felt we had made some major breakthroughs.

When I next saw him, Steven's feet had started to peel. This was also positive as he was *shedding skin*. I mentioned this to him, and he said that's how he felt, as if layers of old emotional issues were being peeled away. The deep ridges in both feet had disappeared in the left foot and were almost gone in the right foot. Instead of being clean, his feet were now a bit grubby. This I felt was also positive as he was starting to 'pick up stuff.'

I continued to see Steven for a few more sessions, during which time, through observing the ever-changing aspects of his feet, we were able to release more of his painful history. The calluses continued to peel off and he was able to establish a closer, more intimate relationship with his girlfriend.

PHYSICAL HEALING

Gently rubbing the callus with pumice stone helps remove layers of these backed up emotions and opens the door to stepping into the future. Dry cracked heels can be both painful and unsightly; when the problem persists, especially for diabetics or people with impaired vascular sufficiency, this can lead to a serious medical problem and it's worth having the situation checked by a podiatrist or doctor.

EMOTIONAL CAUSES

One needs to ask where we have become stuck. Why are you afraid to move ahead? What is holding you back from doing what you want to do? Does your family still govern your life? Is it not time to start living your life the way you want to? What can you do to bring about the desired change?

Cuts

KEY ISSUES
Feeling wounded by a situation or person.

EMOTIONAL CAUSES
My young daughter stood on the edge of a broken mirror and cut open her foot on the area between the ball of her foot (heart area) and upper instep. It was at a time when she was feeling very *cut-up* about a situation at school which was causing her much *heartache*.

Cuts often indicate deep emotional wounds where we may feel angry with ourselves for allowing others to breakthrough our boundaries. A cut occurs as the result of an external object, so the wound is usually to do with another person or situation that threatens us, rather than some internal issue. Wounds bleed which, interestingly enough, comes from *blodam* which means 'that which bursts out." As cuts are sudden and unexpected, it could have to do with a situation or person that has suddenly emerged, or a sudden rush of emotions on our part, about a situation or event, which causes us to bleed.

To get further insight we need to look at exactly where the cut has occurred. Most likely it would be on the underside of either the foot, on the heel - family/groups of people, fear, victim issues; or on the lower instep- relationship, financial, sexual, guilt issues; on the upper instep - self-esteem, anger, our rights; or on the ball of the foot - issues of unresolved grief, intimacy, self-love. This would indicate where or what we are feeling *cut-up* about. Perhaps the situation threatens *to cut us down to size*, or *cut in half*, as in make us feel divided about our loyalties; if it falls on the lower instep, do we need to *cut our losses* financially?

CASE STUDY
Case one: In a shocking case, a nine year-old child was being bullied so badly at school that he developed an ulcer. He also had numerous small cuts on the heart chakra that he complained about constantly, but which never seemed to heal. They bled and *wept profusely*, showing how unbearable his life had become. Fortunately the situation was dealt with, but such deep scars will no doubt remain.

Case two: Sometimes the universe speaks to us very directly, as in this case when a client managed to cut his foot open on my wooden

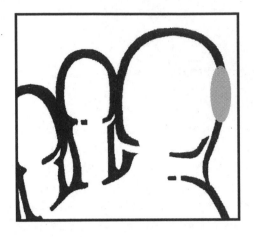

Fig. 40 · Nose cut

massage table, right on the area of the nose reflex. The mystery remains as to how, covered in blankets, he managed to do so. This occurred while we were discussing his need for recognition, which is related to the nose reflex. It was an incredible affirmation that we had touched a deep wound. His need for approval and the lack of that support, was cutting him up and destroying his life and happiness.

HEALING

If a situation is *cutting us up*, the wound will not heal by ignoring it. Like a physical wound it needs to be cleaned out before it can heal. Otherwise it will simply fester. If you have sustained a cut, ask yourself whether someone is trying to *cut you down to size*. Do you need to *cut back* in areas of your life? Does someone need to *cut it out* in terms of their behaviour towards you? Using the exact location of the cut and referring to the chakra concerned will help you to determine more about its cause.

Flat Feet

KEY ISSUES
Support and grounding.

PHYSICAL CAUSES
Everyone has flat feet at birth, mirroring a baby's need for constant support. (Unlike other animal species, it takes human babies far longer before they can survive alone.) Arches develop during childhood and by age 12 or 13 are usually fully developed.

People with flat feet generally feel that they lack support in life or are not supported by those around them – it's like being in that vulnerable baby state when you need to feel constantly supported. Likewise many elderly people suffer from flat feet, as their support system crumbles around them. It is as if the foot collapses (or is drawn down to the earth) in an attempt to feel grounded and supported. And because they may not feel grounded, they may very often have boundary issues.

CASE STUDY
Miriam had a thriving dental practice, and her whole life had focused around her patients, particularly since her divorce, which resulted in her being the sole supporter of two children. Her troubled relationship with both her ex-husband and her children who had problems, had left her self-esteem extremely bruised, so it wasn't hard to see why she would work really hard at her dentistry as, in this area of her life, she felt confident and uplifted. She had high expectations of herself and drove herself relentlessly to meet these. Long hours and years of stress had taken their toll on her health and she was forced to take time off work to allow her body to heal.

Months turned into years and realizing that she would not be able to resume her role and the demands it placed on her she was forced to sell out to a junior partner. Now the practice she had nurtured for so many years was under the control of someone else. The hours she had spent administering healing to others was not reciprocated and she was understandably angry and bitter that now in her moment of need, patients, colleagues and family were not only absent but in some cases avoided her altogether. Over the years she had always felt unsupported but was too busy to acknowledge it. Now with time to herself she realized just how bitter she was. It was not surprising then for me to see that her arches were very flat mirroring the lack of support she felt in life.

PHYSICAL HEALING

There is not much that can be done in the way of conventional treatment, except for exercising and in some cases using shoe inserts.

EMOTIONAL HEALING

We are constantly supported in life, but often we just aren't aware of it. We may also feel we are alone, unsupported and that life is collapsing around us; in fact, it may simply be the end of an era, thus opening the way to the beginning of a new more enjoyable period of our lives. If you are experiencing a period like this in your life, I suggest you lie on the ground or lean against a large tree. Feel its solid comforting support and then acknowledge and affirm that you are being supported on your life journey, even if it's not working out the way you had planned.

Footprints

KEY ISSUES
The impression you make in the world.

OBSERVATIONS
Our footprints are the impression that we leave behind when we walk on our life's path. When celebrities leave their hands and footprints in wet cement outside famous buildings, they leave a lasting impression of themselves. When we take a child's shoe, hand or foot and cast it in bronze or plaster, we attempt to hold onto the memory or impression of them as they were.

Indigenous game trackers can tell simply by looking at an animal's footprint, much about the nature and mental state of their prey. We have lost this art, although by identifying someone's shoes as Nike or Gucci, we can still tell a reasonable amount about a person!

Large footprints, indicate that we could create a big impression in the world, while small footprints indicate our contribution may be more subtle, but no less worthwhile. Sometimes feet will leave a gentle impression, while other feet push hard into the sand. The heavier the imprint, the greater the burden the person may feel they are carrying; alternatively, they may be solid and down-to-earth, or they may even want to dominate situations or people. A faint impression could indicate an airy, up-in-the-clouds, insecure, or even an enlightened person. Notice also what areas of the foot are pressed more deeply into the soil. If the heel leaves a deep imprint while the ball of the foot barely shows, the person could be carrying issues to do with their family, religious community, colleagues or other groups they are associated with. Reversed, there may be issues of the heart that weigh the individual down. One foot may show these aspects more than the other, in which case the burden would have more to do with male (right) and/or past issues, as opposed to female (left) and/or present issues.

If it's the toe prints that are most prominent, the person may be a great thinker, or someone who wants his or her ideas to create a marked impression on the world. If the ridge of the foot is very pronounced, the person may be carrying issues concerning the need to control, while a flat footed imprint may indicate a grounded person or someone who is trying to get grounded.

While walking over the same area, some people can pick up a lot more than others, i.e. their feet get much dirtier. This too is not chance, but rather an indicator of someone's ability to "pick-up" on issues – for instance, how sensitive they are to their environment. A clean foot on someone who has just walked over a floor would indicate that the person does not pick up much around them, while a clean foot which gets dirty walking over the same floor, would indicate extreme sensitivity. I had one client, no matter whether he wore shoes or not, always had pristine clean feet – he was a great guy but not attuned to the sensitivities of those around him, which sometimes drove his wife to distraction.

Some people may have a print where the big toe pushes a bit ahead. This person is either reaching towards the Divine, or wanting to push ahead with new ideas, plans or concepts. A right foot that turns outwards indicates a person who still lives or hankers after the past, while a turned out left foot shows a person who is living ahead of himself or herself, i.e. in the future. If both footprints turn in, the person may be withdrawing or afraid to *get out there*. We speak of people who are duck-footed when both their feet splay outwards. These may be people who are very much united to their families or communities, or who want to be noticed by their family.

Try walking in someone else's footprints. You may be able to pick up much about the person. Next time you take a stroll to the beach then, you can put your skills to the test and discover more about your fellow walkers!

Heel Spurs

KEY ISSUES
Immobility. Fear of taking action in spite of wanting to do so. Holding onto the past.

PHYSICAL CAUSES
Heel spurs are pointed bony outgrowths of the back of the heel (Achilles tendonitis) or on the sole in the region of the heel bone (plantar fascia). The plantar fascia is a fibrous band of connective tissue that runs lengthways on the sole of the foot from the heel to the toes. The bony outgrowth may be as a result of calcification that occurs where the tendon joins the heel bone, as a result of the plantar fascia being inflamed for a long period of time. A sharp thorn-like spur or bone develops and although the spur as such may not be painful, the inflammation around the area on the plantar fascia causes an ache which may be interspersed with a sharp stabbing pain on the heel which will make walking very painful. The pain is often worse after a period of sitting or sleeping.

Inflammation can also occur as a result of a sports injury or from an inflammatory disease (such as arthritis and Ankylosing Spondylitis), or from obesity creating an excessive pressure on the foot, or during pregnancy where one's weight increases dramatically over a short period of time. Also, frequent exercise after a long period of little or no exercise and over-pronation (where the foot rolls inwards) can all be major contributing factors.

EMOTIONAL CAUSES
As the word 'spur' indicates, we need to spur ourselves forward - to move from the known and experience the unknown. Perhaps that is why heel spurs are so common amongst sports people who constantly have to push themselves, or spur themselves onwards to achieve their goals. With people who are overweight, the spurs may be a result of needing to push oneself to get going when one is lethargic and it is hard to find the energy to do so. The calcification is an indication that we are calcified, i.e. our ability to move ahead has become thwarted and we may feel stuck. The formation of spurs shows just how rooted we are to the ground we are currently stand on. No amount of pain, physical or emotional, can shift us. For someone who has not exercised

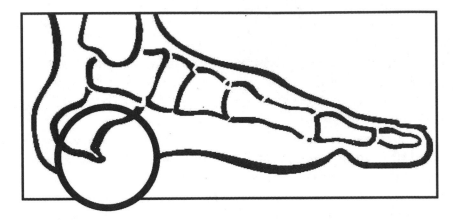

Fig. 41 · Heel spurs

in a long time, spurring oneself to do so may be extremely hard when one has become comfortable with the pleasure of being idle.

CASE STUDY

To most people, it would appear that Janet had it all - a beautiful home, money, friends, a wide variety of interests, a devoted husband, beautiful possessions and children who were reasonably civilized. Yet, when she came to see me, I felt she was searching for a deeper meaning in her life. Her life appeared full and yet I discovered it was spiritually empty. Her relationships were superficial, and a very controlling partner made her afraid and uncertain as to how to make any changes in her life. She was also very self-conscious about the amount of weight that she was carrying.

At first she displayed a reluctance to proceed with the session, feeling that little could really be achieved in terms of her life issues. I could sense her fear of the process and so did my best to relax her.

My overall impression of her feet was their whiteness. I asked if she was feeling run down and she said "no'. This confused me because I had seldom seen such white feet. She had very deep ridges along her feet in the instep (second and third chakras). The ridges were more like cracks in their depth and were more prolific on the right foot. I asked if relationships had been difficult for her and she replied they had. This clearly caused her emotional discomfort and she was reluctant to go into this topic.

Janet had well-formed calluses on her heel and I explained the significance of these in terms of the difficulty with moving ahead, particularly in regard to first chakra issues of security. She then mentioned that she had had spurs removed off both feet.

When I suggested Janet's spurs could also relate to her ability to move in life, she acknowledged that moving forward and changing was not easy for her. It was then that I realized what the whiteness on her feet represented - it was more to do with a feeling of hopelessness and disillusionment with a situation she felt unable to change, than physical exhaustion as such. She immediately related deeply to this suggestion. In this way perhaps her comfort level was more of a hindrance than help. When life does not force us to, we seldom are inclined to change. That is why sometimes our angels have to create a major upheaval, not to hurt us, but to force us into a process of change that can heal us on a deeper level.

PHYSICAL HEALING

Heel spurs are treated in various ways to decrease the associated inflammation and avoid re-injury. Applications of ice helps to reduce pain and inflammation, as does anti-inflammatory medication. Shoe inserts are used to take pressure off the spurs, and heellifts can reduce stress on the Achille's tendon to relieve painful spurs at the back of the heel. Surgery is performed only when the spurs are chronically inflamed.

EMOTIONAL HEALING

Ask where you are afraid to move? What do you perceive is holding you back? Do you want to remain in the same situation forever? You need to take the first step in making a shift. It may be scary but would you rather remain in this position?

Gout

KEY ISSUES

Rigid thoughts. Inability to release past issues. Anger.

PHYSICAL CAUSES

Gout is a disease of the whole body, rather than just the area(s) where it gives pain - most commonly the big toe and occasionally in the ankle joint. Uric acid builds up in the joints, causing inflammation, extreme sensitivity and swelling, which results in pain and discomfort. This condition can develop for two reasons. Firstly, the liver may produce more uric acid than the body can excrete in the urine or secondly, a diet of rich foods (e.g., red meat, cream sauces, red wine) puts more uric acid into the bloodstream than the kidneys can filter. This rich diet is why it has sometimes been referred to as the 'gentlemen's disease.' Over time, the uric acid that should have been flushed away by the kidneys crystallizes and settles into the spaces between the joints. Gout develops quickly and usually only occurs in one joint at a time.

EMOTIONAL CAUSES

These crystals represent the emotions that should have been flushed out by the kidneys. Instead, they build up to the point where they solidify. This implies then that we have become stuck emotionally in past issues and, as the big toe is the primary location, it is our thoughts or thinking about these emotional issues, which we can't release or express. Being in the toe, gout makes it painful to walk or move ahead in our lives and instead we have to remain with our leg up, glued to the spot. Gout is more common in the elderly, who may find it harder to change a fixed way of thinking. This is also why a change of diet is often not adhered to. The gout sufferer finds change hard - and in this area they are not alone!

The swollen and inflamed joint indicates that there is retained anger connected with one's ideas or thinking. The resulting inflexibility reflects not only rigid thinking, but also a desire to rule or be in charge. There may be only one way of thinking that is acceptable – and that's the way of the gout sufferer. Yet, if we suffer from gout, we must have compassion for ourselves or other gout sufferers, by understanding that the need to hold tight to our/their ideas comes only from a deep fear or insecurity that we may be wrong. The fear of letting go and embracing new ideas or change is far greater than the pain their current thinking is causing them.

We must also take into account the cause of the acid buildup, namely alcohol and rich food. Drinking too much may be one way of letting go and it also may be a way of escaping the insecurities that haunt the gout sufferer. Rich foods relate to a desire to feed the lack of emotional richness we feel in our lives. We overindulge as a way to compensate for the lack of love and nurturance we experience in life.

ORIGIN OF WORD

Gout derives from the Old French *gote,* and the Latin *gutta* meaning "drop." The disease was thought to be caused by drops of viscous humors seeping from the blood into the joints, which turned out to be close to the truth. We say when *we hit rock bottom* we land in the gutter (*gutta*). In gout, it is as if all our excesses have dropped to our extremities. We have forgone the subtle and sought refuge in the gross. As such all our repressed anger and rigidity has caused us to *drop out* from actively embracing life and continue to drop back into old habits.

CASE STUDY

Having read the nature of a gout sufferer in terms of the ability to adapt to new ways of thinking, it will probably not come as a huge surprise to find out that I have never had a person with gout come to see me! The only example then I can use is that of a friend's partner, who recently developed gout. He was a portly man who enjoyed copious quantities of fine red wine and plenty of rich food (before the onset of gout that is). Having to forego these pleasures was hard, and I suspect not always adhered to! In appearance he bore the typical look of a gentleman who enjoyed indulgences - a swollen, puffy face, wide pores and red nose, together with that pallid aura of unhealthiness that accompanies those who do not exercise or see enough sunlight. He was, as his interests showed, a great chef who enjoyed cooking up a storm for his guests.

For most of his working life he had been employed by the same firm, doing the same job. Whilst appearing contented in the office, at home he would fume about the situation that he found himself in. No matter how poorly he was treated, resigning was simply never an option, in spite of being financially sound enough to cope with being unemployed. Hoarding was also a passion - anything from old electrical cables, to radio parts, to strange culinary ingredients (long past expiry date), or fishing equipment a sport he spent rather more time talking about than actually doing.

It was clear though that there were many issues in his past that he had not dealt with - in particular those stemming from a rigid upbringing. His way of coping with any difficult emotional situation was to withdraw into a fuming silence. For all this, he was a kindly, generous man, with a great love of animals and he was a loving husband.

His partner had had a great love prior to meeting him and she still held deep feelings for her ex-lover. It must be hard to cope with a situation when you are aware that your partner still loves someone else. Unable to plumb the depths of his unexpressed emotions, or in any way to change his life, he settled, understandably, for rich food and drink, rather that the richness of relationship or spirit.

One can only feel compassion for this man caught up in the painful web of his own creation, yet feeling unable to move beyond it.

PHYSICAL HEALING

If an excess of uric acid in the joint is the cause of the pain, decreasing it can bring about a speedy relief. Introducing a healthy, alkaline diet will do wonders, which means red wine and steak dinners will be a thing of the past! Doctors will frequently report that it is hard to alter the eating/drinking habits of the gout sufferer (no doubt as a result of past rigid patterns of thinking), and consequently the disease will recur with increasing regularity.

EMOTIONAL HEALING

Whom do you need to forgive - yourself or someone else? What issues do you still hold onto from the past? Why are you afraid to change your thinking? How would you feel if your thoughts were wrong? Would you rather remain rigid? To be flexible means the ability to grow; rigidity holds you in the past. Are you trying to replace spiritual emptiness with physical richness?

Hammer Toes

KEY ISSUES

Thinking or intellectual input/insights suppressed. Feeling that others are hammering your ideas and beliefs. Afraid to stand tall. Holding back thoughts for fear of offending.

PHYSICAL CAUSES

When ligaments and tendons in the foot tighten, toes contract at the middle joint causing the toe's joints to curl downwards. Hammer toes (of which there are two types, flexible and rigid) can occur in all toes except the big toe. The flexible hammer toe can be straightened manually, whereas attempting to move the rigid hammer toe can be very painful. There is often discomfort at the top part of the toe as it rubs against the shoe, resulting in corns or calluses.

EMOTIONAL CAUSES

Hammer toes are fairly common with the advance of bunions and further represent the sufferer's ideas and thoughts of being literally hammered on by others. There may be intellectual abuse causing tension and the desire to pull back or bow down to someone else's point of view, simply to maintain peace. Not standing up to others also affects our self-esteem, particularly if the hammer toe is the third toe (relationship to self); if the second toe is affected, this relates to our feelings and not speaking up for ourselves within our family or at work. The fourth toe relates to holding back from exploring our ideas and thoughts about money, sex and relationships and it relates to security issues if the baby toe is hammered.

Sometimes the actual tops of the toe pads have small indents that look as if someone has taken a small hammer to them. This relates to having our ideas knocked on the head by others or ourselves as a result of a need for perfection.

CASE STUDY

Case one: Martha was a personal assistant to the managing director of a retail chain. She was in her early forties and had a trim, athletic figure, which she enhanced by being a personal fitness coach after hours. She had divorced and remarried, although this second marriage also had its difficulties, as her husband had been unemployed for most of

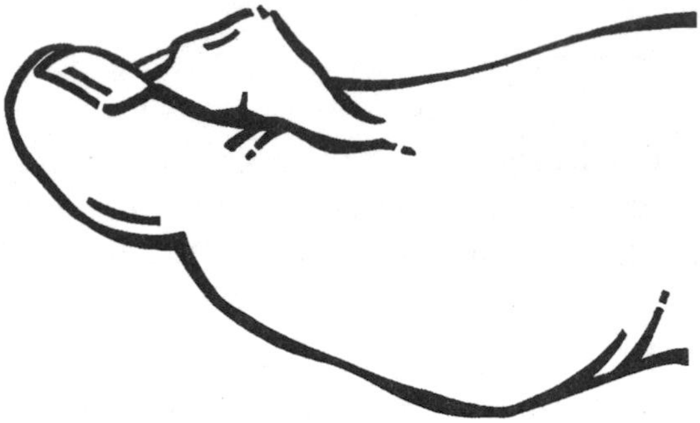

Fig. 42 · Hammer Toe

their time together. Adding to her stressful relationship, were her two teenage daughters who, at the ages of 22 and 17, did not enjoy living at home, but were unable to earn sufficient money to live independently. This caused further friction in the home.

Yellow calluses on the heart reflexes on both feet mirrored how extremely fed up or resentful she felt with her marriage.

The tops of all her toes were dented, and the toes themselves appeared to have been pushed back into their sockets. While the right toes were straight, the third, fourth and fifth toes on the left foot were scrunched up. I asked her if she ever felt like her thoughts or ideas were knocked or dented by those around her. She said her mother in particular was scornful of her new spiritual approach to life. Noticing that the necks of the toes were constricted, particularly on the left side, I followed this further by asking if she felt it difficult to express what she felt to her mother. She said she did. Whereas in the past she had often lost her temper and told her mother just what she thought, she didn't do so now for fear of hurting or upsetting the old lady, which could lead to further health complications. We then talked about how this was blocking not just her expression to her mother, but her ability to express her emotions in general. Also by subtly giving off this message of "Don't speak your truth or anything offensive to me or you might kill me," the mother had found a wonderfully manipulative tool.

A mother who feels disempowered and/or has low self-esteem may seek to control her daughter by withdrawing approval that the daughter then constantly tries to gain. When this occurs, we mustn't blame the mother, but rather have compassion for her insecurity and fear that manifested as control. At the same time though, we can choose not to play the game by seeking approval from ourselves only.

In examining vulnerability and her family, Martha spoke at length about her daughters who fought with her husband, each wanting to assume control. She felt constantly trapped between them and frequently tried to rescue the situation, although she was aware that she was not helping by doing this. Deep grooves on both feet on the instep at the first and second chakras demonstrated the problems she was having. I mentioned the scattered lines and diagonal crossed lines all over the insteps and suggested that the situation might make her feel confused and unsure of what direction to take. She agreed.

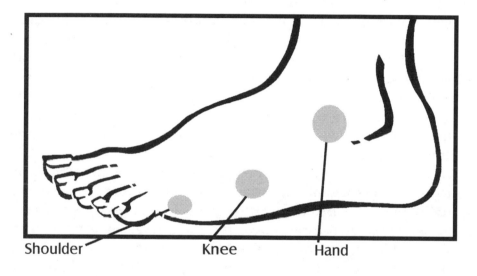

Shoulder   Knee   Hand

Fig. 43 · Outside of foot

The tops of her feet showed a strong need for perfection. She related to this and to the amount of pressure she put on herself because of it. Bony ridges indicated her need for structure, and were no doubt the reason she made a good PA. Her hand reflex was also very flat and I asked her just how much she ever acknowledged her own achievements, or did she just carry on doing without ever celebrating? She related to these questions and became very emotional.

Afterwards she said that at one point during our session she had felt as if she could not breathe and she had felt energy shooting up her legs. I then asked her if at times she felt as if she was trapped and she replied that her mother in particular made her feel like she was She said she also felt that way with her children, as well as being in the situation of the prime breadwinner. She came to the conclusion that she needed to start living her own life and not try to be everything to everyone else.

In Martha's case, we have all aspects of hammered toes: her beliefs, feelings and thoughts repressed by her mother, and to an extent by her daughters and her husband; she felt fearful of standing up to them all, and so suppressed her own thoughts for fear of offending her family.

In conclusion, Martha was one of those wonderful clients who proceeded to put a great deal of effort into making changes in her life. She said that experiencing a foot treatment had been one of the most amazing experiences of her life. Apparently, after having spent some time in nature in order to process all that had happened, she then went home and cracked open a bottle of champagne to celebrate all she had achieved in her life! Forgetting the need for perfection, she had allowed herself to let her hair down, much to the surprise of her family, who were irritated that she was not bowing to their needs. She subsequently made a concerted effort to create boundaries with her mother and continued to gain confidence in her own belief structure.

Case two: One client, who suffered from hammered toes, was constantly being ridiculed by her extremely intelligent, but low-achieving spouse. While he refused to find employment, he resented her success, particularly because her career involved socializing. Her achievements only created further tension, as he sought to level the playing fields by what amounted to verbal abuse. Any suggestion she came up with, from a dinner dish to a home improvement, was met with contempt. Her desire to please him came about because he had made her feel guilty of her success, a manipulative tool that his martyr archetype reveled in.

Case three: Another client came to me with hammer toes, in particular the second toes. She had been rejected by both parents and brought up by her grandmother. Grandma's own children, who were still quite young, resented her intrusion into their lives and made her life intolerable. As a young child this rejection must have badly affected her sense of self-esteem. She saw her mother sporadically over the years, and was well into her fifties before she finally met her father. The belief that her parents had not loved her sufficiently to keep her, was a belief that was to make a devastating imprint on her life. The lack of self love was represented on toes that were squashed i.e. no one had room/time for her. She learnt to repress her thoughts and feelings so as not to offend anyone.

As an adult, in her job she still could not express emotions and thoughts for fear of them being rejected. So she constantly held herself back, yet resented her lack of career advancement, and had virtually become a "Yes-man." She was often stressed about her job and imagined that others found her contribution worthless. Her intelligence was overlooked and promotion constantly passed her by. It was definitely understandable why her toes were as hammered as she felt.

PHYSICAL HEALING

Hammer toes may seem like minor irritations but, if left untreated, they become serious permanent deformities. Calluses can form, usually on the tops of the toes and ulcers may develop. When deformities reach this stage, the toes are fixed in a bent position and cannot be easily straightened. For this reason, it is important to obtain treatment for the toes before they become fixed.

When the toes first start to buckle, they can be straightened easily and if flat feel cause the problem, a podiatrist can fit the patient for custom-molded shoe inserts that provide a better arch for the foot and help the muscles work together. In these cases, the prognosis is good. Without treatment, the soft tissue structures that attach to hammer toes begin to tighten and a rigid deformity results. Surgery is then necessary either to lengthen a shortened toe muscle or in more serious cases, a variety of progressive procedures may be used. If these fail, one final procedure that may restore normal mobility involves fusing two bones together.

EMOTIONAL HEALING

To overcome hammer toes one needs to stop losing energy over what others think. So many great ideas never see the light of day because we share them with someone who belittles them. We tell someone we want to start a company and before we have even finished speaking they have told us we lack the skill/qualifications/contacts/finances etc. to do the job. Unsure of ourselves, we are convinced by the end of the conversation that they are right and so we never explore our potential. If people who hammer your thinking surround you, stop communicating your ideas with them. You don't need their approval to proceed (unless of course you are a minor). Let your ideas take flight. You'll never know until you try, and there is no such thing as failure. If others are offended by your potential, then it is their issues not yours that are the problem. No one has the right to suppress your potential.

High Arches

KEY ISSUES
Perfectionism.

PHYSICAL CAUSES
High arches can be a hereditary condition and can also occur should the muscles in the foot contract due to an underlying neurological or muscular problem. They can also be a normal variant just as some people have longer toes etc. There is some thought that highheeled shoes may exacerbate or even cause some instances of high arches. The arch raises high off the ground and sometimes the heel may tilt inwards and this can be accompanied by clawed toes.

EMOTIONAL CAUSES
"Limited range of motion and doesn't absorb shock (change) well," is how a running shoe manufacturer referred in his advertising brochure to people with high arched or rigid feet. Inadvertently they also described the emotional make-up of those people. When we have high arches, it reveals that we are perfectionists who put a lot of pressure on ourselves to get things right. In our need to be perfect, we also become rigid in the way we think – we have set ways of doing things and it is hard to change those ideas. Life is all about change, so this can make it a painful experience when we strive to remain static in a changing and imperfect world, even though it can be said that it's only our perception that sees the world as imperfect. Very pronounced ridges of bone on the top of the foot towards the toes, indicate that we are also people who are entrenched in the need for structure. Unlike flat-footed people this rigidity may result in boundaries that make us addicted to security and resistant to change. Being "higher" make us appear arrogant and removed or aloof.

CASE STUDY
Jill was sent to see me by her mother who was concerned about her daughter. When I started working with her I was aware of her sunken adrenal glands, the whiteness of her feet and the lacklustre dry skin on her soles. It was clear that she was exhausted and burnt out. She had two children under the age of three and worked mornings only. Understandably she was exhausted, but many women maintain a similar lifestyle without a complete depletion of energy. (I have to say that, at

that same period in my life, I wasn't exactly a ball of fire!) Jill's high arches, however, indicated that the problem might be more than just the stresses of motherhood.

I asked Jill if she was a perfectionist. She laughed and said she was. Everything had to be just right and it was causing her endless frustration to have her children mess up what she had just tidied; toys were constantly pulled out and spread all over the place; clothes were removed from where Jill had put them away, and strewn happily around. She felt she could not be happy unless her house was 100% in order. The obvious impossibility of this goal made her frustrated and resentful towards her husband, who appeared unconcerned about the accumulation of debris and who, in fact, added to it.

Jill realized as we spoke that her desire for a perfect house was more a desire that she herself be perfect. I spoke about perfectionism being an unrealistic illusion, as for something to be perfect it must surely be complete. Nothing in the world or in the divine is complete – we are all, and everything around us, in a constant state of evolving. A day ends, but a new one begins; the flower dies but its seeds sprout anew. To expect that she should be perfect then was not only unrealistic but illusionary. Also by whose standards was she judging this lack of perfection? My idea of perfect may differ widely from yours - a perfect meal for me may consist of homemade pasta and a simple but exciting sauce. You may loathe pasta and opt for a tender steak. Which of us chooses the perfect meal?

Through this discussion with Jill, she came to see just how much pressure this issue was causing her not to mention the unhappy atmosphere in the home. She decided to allow her standards to drop a few notches and utilize the time she would save by pampering herself. She started to play with her children as opposed to scolding them.

HEALING

Various footwear inserts are available to help alleviate the pain that might occur from high arches. However on an emotional level the message is: Let go. Ease up. Stop setting unrealistic goals that leave you feeling down when you don't achieve them. Realise people will love you for who you are rather than how perfect you or your surroundings appear.

Ingrown Toenails

KEY ISSUES

Seeking protection. Feeling vulnerable. Self-doubt. Insecurity regarding one's ideas or thoughts.

PHYSICAL CAUSES

An ingrown toenail occurs when the skin on the side of the nail grows over the edge of the nail or when the nail curls and grows into the skin. This can be caused by a number of factors including arthritis, where the toes themselves curl, driving the nail inwards; stubbing one's toe or having it stepped on can cause some of the nail to push into the skin; very large toenails on smaller toes; running in ill-fitting shoes; incorrect cutting of the nails (when they are not cut straight across the top); or occasionally on bedridden patients where bedsheets are tucked in tightly and consequently cause pressure on the toes.

Often, because of the warm, moist environment a bacterial infection can develop, causing red and inflamed skin around the nail, which untreated can cause a severe infection. Watch for swelling, pain, inflammation or a discharge, all of which indicate an infection has set in. Podiatrists will then trim or remove the infected nail or a portion of the overgrown skin. In the case of a re-occurrence, the podiatrist may decide to remove (with a chemical solution) some of the nail that actually grows in the nail bed, making the nail narrower and less inclined to curl inwards. If infected, this procedure may not be possible and the entire nail may need to be removed.

EMOTIONAL CAUSES

Our toe-nails are our toes' protection. The toes are like antennae that pick-up thoughts and ideas from the outside world, as well as, through their rigidity, backing up our own concepts, thoughts or ideas when we need to express them. Remember that the toes are representative of our heads and the nails consequently act as shields for them. On the hands, nails play more of an attacking/defensive role, as we use them to claw and scratch when in a fighting situation.

When toe nails grow in they often curl on the sides and resemble a tortoise shell. Crawling back into our shell is similar to how we feel when we develop ingrowing toenails. If an infection develops, it shows that we feel as if we are at war or odds with a situation.

ORIGIN OF WORD

Inflammation has origins from *flamma* or flame, which in turn relates to fire and anger. The toxins and the body's resistance are indeed engaged in battle over the *inflammatory* situation. For there to be a war, there needs to be an enemy. So whenever there is inflammation, there will be a perceived enemy, whom we feel is violating us. Being on the toes, this will relate specifically to a general attack on our ideas and thoughts.

If the **big toe** has the ingrown toenail, then we could narrow that down to ideas/thoughts/concepts specifically related to spirituality, intuition, our insights, visions, creativity and communication that we doubt or feel vulnerable about. If the **second toe** (the one next to the big toe relating to chakra 4) has the ingrown toenail, then perhaps we are creating a shield or questioning our thoughts and emotions regarding nurturing, love, self-love and grief. When the **third toe** has an ingrown toenail, maybe we are protecting or questioning the thoughts we have regarding our own self-confidence, energy and individuation; while the **second toe** relates to questioning our thoughts about personal power, sexuality, guilt, relationship and financial issues, or feeling others are attacking those thoughts. An ingrown **little toe** nail would indicate uncertainty about our beliefs regarding fear, family and security.

CASE STUDY

Case One: Being a teenager is not easy. There are insecurities, emotional mood swings and the awkwardness of exploring one's sexuality in a repressed society. For a sensitive young man, these issues can become even more problematic and such was the case with Tim, a very artistic and musically talented young man who, in a single sex school where rugby and jocks rule supreme, was bullied.

Tim had beautiful feet - long and graceful with extremely long toes, which mirrored his creative ability. He spent many hours a week playing his violin and hoped to become a professional musician when he finished school. He had an ingrown toenail on the big toe of his right foot, indicating that the issues involved had to do with boys or men. The nail had been treated previously, but had now reappeared, although there had been no specific trigger.

With his long toes, Tim clearly had the potential to be highly creative, yet expressed frustration at his ideas not being met with approval from his peers. This made him question his ideas and in many instances doubt their validity. Consequently he would fall in with the pack in order not to be singled out and become the victim of derision. His second toes were longer than his big toes, which indicated that, given the opportunity, he had the potential to lead with his unique ideas. The frustration at not feeling free to express them hindered his ability to advance, even while keeping him safe. We spoke about how it is those with the ability to think differently that in the end succeed in life, not necessarily those who are six feet tall and can tackle well in football. He needed to trust his ideas and follow them through and not feel so threatened constantly if he was to succeed in establishing his own unique identity.

Case Two: Doris had thickened and ingrown toenails on both her big toes, caused she felt from having to hide her thoughts and beliefs about her spiritual beliefs from her Calvinistic family. Having lived alone for much of her life, Doris had developed an interest in the spiritual aspects of life, something not commonly followed by the majority of people, particularly in her community. Her ingrown toenails came as a result of having to constantly defend her ideas against the scrutiny of others. This caused her to doubt her chosen path, when others logic of others seemed to ridicule her thoughts. She often did not say what she truly thought for fear of the negative reaction of others, yet it angered her that she could not say what she truly believed.

PHYSICAL HEALING

Preparations can be obtained that harden the skin and shrink the soft tissue next to the nail. Soaking in warm soapy or salt water, followed by thorough drying and the application of a mild antiseptic together with a bandage may help the uninfected toe. However, for an infected toe medical advice should be sought.

EMOTIONAL HEALING

If we feel that others are attacking our ideas and thoughts, then we need to look at developing our inner confidence to the point that we do not seek approval of others before moving ahead. We need to trust that if we have the thought, we have been given the idea because we have the capability to carry it forward. Thwarting this process stops us from achieving our awesome potential. For an idea to be made manifest, it requires vision, communication, our heartfelt efforts, self-confidence, financial and/or energy before it can be given birth. Ask yourself where you are inhibiting your ideas? Who makes you question your thoughts? Why do you allow them to do so?

Nails - thickening

KEY ISSUES

Protection of thoughts. Strength to stick with ideas/ thoughts. Protect our intuitive insights.

PHYSICAL CAUSES

Sometimes a fungal or bacterial infection can be the cause of thickened nails, which can then also split, and become disfigured or discoloured. Sometimes the nails can become so thick that they cause pain when they press against other toes or the inside of shoes. Patients with **diabetes** are prone to develop thickened nails, because blood circulation is poor in the extremities, and the body's ability to fight infections is compromised.

EMOTIONAL CAUSES

As has been previously mentioned, our nails protect our toes and consequently our ideas and thoughts. Any deformity, thickening or abnormality of the nails should be viewed with this in mind. To get more specific we need to look at the individual chakras to see what those thoughts and ideas relate to.

If a **nail splits**, it could indicate we are split as to what to do when it comes to a thought or idea. If the nail has **torn**, are we feeling torn apart by a thought or having to defend it, or do we feel vulnerable at having our ideas torn from us? **White spots** on the nail are often an indication of having had a health issue. Obviously having **no nail** would leave us feeling very exposed and tender.

Where there is a **thickening of the nail**, it is an indication that the person needs extra protection. Perhaps he or she feels that others want to hammer their ideas, as in the following examples:

CASE STUDY

Case One: On Joan's right foot there was a large callus on the top of her fourth toe (second chakra), as well as a thickened nail. This area of her foot was red, and almost flashing for my attention. I spoke to her about the significance of a thickened nail, as well as calluses. Falling in the second chakra indicated that the issue potentially lay with close relationships, partnerships, as well as money etc. She agreed to being very vulnerable in this area and experiencing great anger towards her partner, who had lost his job some time ago and who appeared to be doing little to find another. He had also rejected her sexually (fourth toe) which added to her frustration, as showed by the red and inflamed toe. He also was inclined to drink heavily and could become verbally abusive when intoxicated. No wonder she needed some protection!

Case Two: Carol had thickened nails on both her small toes. Protection she felt from a very hectic family environment. Mother of two teenage sons and a very demanding husband who she referred to as a third child, she found herself constantly suppressing her needs for the sake of theirs. Her husband would even refer to her as "Mummy," when addressing her, compounding his belief in his wife as the nurturing mother to him the needy, naughty child. Any ideas she had relating to changing the family setup, such as getting the boys to assist with chores, were met with ridicule. She was frustrated and disillusioned with life, and had come to see me primarily because of a painful knee.

There were also very noticeable calluses on her pineal/pituitary reflexes and I suggested that sometimes this happens when we block off our guidance. She asked me why we might do that and I replied that sometimes our guidance tells us what we don't want to hear, so it becomes safer to close down or desensitize this area. She said she could understand that and then asked how she could learn to stand up for herself – to fight against the suppression she felt instead of denying or complying with it. After further discussion I said I felt she had great potential to develop other interests besides being a mother, as she was bright, creative and had an obvious flair for interior design, and there was still time to explore other avenues. I then worked silently on her feet before moving up and concentrating via Reiki on her knee. As Carol received the Reiki treatment, she became deeply relaxed and as I worked I felt a tremendous release. Later she said that the knee was no longer painful. To counteract her fear of its reoccurrence I suggested she take a look at her own need to be nurtured and start actively making all her "children" more independent. This would free the way for her to move ahead with ease.

PHYSICAL HEALING

Thickened nails can be difficult to treat because nails grow slowly and receive very little blood supply. However, there have been recent advances in treatment options, including oral and topical medications, but they should not be taken by patients with liver disease. If in doubt consult your doctor. Because nails grow very slowly, it typically takes 6 months to a year for the nail to regain a healthy, clear, thin appearance.

EMOTIONAL HEALING

First we need to ascertain what or whom we feel we need to protect ourselves from. Then we can start the process of confronting instead of avoiding the issues involved. When we build a wall, we not only shut others out, but we also shut ourselves in, making it hard to connect intimately with others. We can become hardened not only to others, but also to our own needs. Interestingly, in both the previous cases, the women were well rounded, indicating that they a) they were carrying the weight of their unhappiness and b) the extra layer of skin was another way of shielding themselves from others. *Weight* makes us inclined to *wait* before we do anything – we become stuck in our own unhappy situations. Sometimes we have to let go of our protection if we are to get ahead.

Skin Peeling

KEY ISSUES
Shedding of the old. Renewal. Release.

PHYSICAL CAUSES
The type of peeling skin that is being referred to is not that which is caused by a fungal infection, such as Athlete's Foot, psoriasis or as a result of taking certain medicines. Rather it occurs spontaneously and causes no pain, redness or other side effect and once having peeled does not continue to do so.

EMOTIONAL CAUSES
The night before I knew that my husband's business would have to close, I recall having a dream of my feet about to peel. In the dream, I was at the doctor's office, unsure if there was some sort of fungal infection, or if the feet were simply peeling naturally. In the dream I was afraid of the skin peeling away, as the layer was very thick and would leave my skin raw and exposed, making walking painful.

The question was whether it was something alien that was getting *under my skin,* such as something attacking me/us, or simply a natural peeling away of old layers, as we both shifted and grew. Did my response require a warrior-type approach or simply an acceptance of the natural evolvement of our lives?

Another dream a few days later gave me further clues; I saw the whole under-sole about to peel away, making me afraid of how painful it would feel to step forward in life as my skin was now raw and exposed. The rawness of the exposed foot mirrored my own vulnerability and the pain I felt at having to move on from this setback. Yet it was in truth not a setback, but a shedding of an old way of life, one that I had clung onto rather too dearly!

Whenever we shed skin we shed the outer layer of our being, because the skin is like a large screen onto which we project our inner emotional and physical life. Someone with deathly pallid skin is seldom healthy. Equally, all the skin eruptions, blushes and blemishes that appear, are a reminder of what is happening within us. When the skin peels away, either in one chakra or over the whole foot, it's an indication that the past is being shed. It is the sloughing off of the old to make way for the new.

CASE STUDY

Petra had decided after a number of years to have a baby. She had a top job in an advertising agency and was well- respected in her field. The company she worked for made it clear they would not tolerate her being unable to work late and entertain clients because of the baby; it was all or nothing and that she would have to make that decision. Once the baby was born and the three months of official maternity leave had passed, Petra tried to resume her job. She was miserable. Disturbed sleep, the pressure of work, and the emotional trauma each time she had to leave her baby brought her close to having a breakdown. Instead she had a breakthrough and made the decision to leave her job.

Not without some sense of regret, Petra made the move from boardroom to babyroom. Shortly after the move, the skin on both feet peeled off entirely, indicating her physical and emotional shift. (See also Steven's case history under Corns and calluses.)

HEALING

Letting go and embracing change is part of how we move and grow in life. Change is constant, yet we insist on getting angry when it happens and continue clinging to the past. Whenever we make a change, we so often presume that it will be for the worst and yet it seldom is. How many people do you know who have lost their jobs only to find a new way of making a living which makes them far happier.

Shoes

KEY ISSUES
Protection. How we ground ourselves. How we proceed in life.

PHYSICAL CAUSES
The need to protect our feet stretches way back in history. In fact a sandal was discovered in Missouri in America, dating back to 6000 BC. I suspect that were it not for the relative fragility of the materials that made up our ancestors' footwear, such as leather, plant materials, etc., even earlier examples might have survived. Sandals seem to have been the most popular shoes worn in ancient civilizations; however, a few early cultures did make more closed-in, moccasin-type shoes. Interestingly enough, it has only been in the last two hundred years that pairs of shoes were made that were not identical, i.e. the left foot differing from the right foot.

As man developed so the emphasis switched from shoes being purely protective, to being an outward display of his/her social and financial position. (They were not necessarily made with comfort in mind if we recall stiletto heels; or in the Middle Ages there was the Crackow, with a toe length of around 12cm; and then in the 15th century the Chopine appeared which was over 90cms high and the wearer required a servant on either side simply to maintain balance!). If *clothes maketh the man*, then shoes certainly served to enhance or elevate status, hence the popularity of high heels. In short, you are what you wear. Or as the old saying goes, "Don't judge another until you've walked a mile in his shoes/moccasins."

EMOTIONAL ISSUES
Symbolically, our shoes represent how we go through life. They indicate the steps we take. If they are worn but comfortable, then comfort rather than lavish luxury is clearly where we are at. When we buy new shoes, we open up the gateway to a new way of walking our lives, much the same way as a new hairstyle or car would do.

We often slip into our shoes without thinking about them. They have become such a familiar part of our wardrobe that we no longer are aware of them.

Here is an exercise to get you more in touch with your shoes and yourself:

Select the shoes you wear most often. It can be one or several pairs.

Spend some time examining them and write down your first impression of them. My shoes are... Worn and scruffy? Are they more worn on the left or right foot? Smart and newly polished? Trendy? Flamboyant? Muted? Made to last? Comfortable? Cheap even though you can afford better? Colourful? Expensive even though you cannot really afford them? Falling to pieces? Uncomfortable? Smelly? Pristine? Broken? And so on.

Now look carefully at what you have written and, as you did in Chapter Three, replace the words "my shoes" with "I am." For instance if you have written: "My shoes are comfortable, but well worn." You would write "I am comfortable, but well worn." Ask yourself then if you are feeling worn out? Are you comfortable with your life? Or has comfort become complacency?

If you wrote "cheap" ask yourself if you really nurture yourself or, if you give freely to others, do you do little for yourself? If they are uncomfortable but you wear them anyhow, in what areas of your life are you experiencing uncomfortable situations which you choose to ignore or sweep under the carpet?

Are the heels worn down? Do you feel down at heel, tired of living with lack? Or do you have high heels that make you feel well-heeled or powerful and wealthy? If the left heel is more worn than the right then perhaps you feel that women or female duties to do with the family are tiresome and tiring. If the right sole is more worn, then is something from the past or a male/your own inner male, wearing you thin? Just being aware of what your shoes look and feel like will give you insight into how you feel about yourself.

THE TYPES OF SHOES WE WEAR AND WHY

Walk into someone's home and you have an instant insight into what sort of person they might be. Shoes are no different in revealing something about the wearer.

Here are a few examples:

STILETTOS

It is completely illogical to wear stiletto shoes! They squish the toes together painfully and the angle of the ankle is not only precarious but bad for your posture and back. They are also said to cause bunions and other foot related problems. Yet stilettos still remain popular.

If you love to wear high stilettos, what you are really seeking is to be higher than men – to raise yourselves above them. You want to become a goddess to be worshipped and adored; to walk tall; to lead and not to follow. You are the out-of-reach seductress, beautiful, but unobtainable (unless as a man, you have the ability to obtain height or status financially).

INDUSTRIAL BOOTS, DOCKERS ETC.

The heavy industrial look of these boots lets other people be aware of the fact that the wearer is not to be taken lightly. It's incongruous to wear these hot, heavily heeled boots when the closest you are going to get to a safari, is a walk to the nearest fish and chip shop. Yet young men, so commonly emasculated by women, need to verify their masculinity in some way. Given their tough appearance, these boots convey the hardcore personality their wearer would like to have. Women too like to wear boots , often in striking contrast to feminine skirts. The message here is simple: I'm a woman but that doesn't mean you can mess with me.

COLOURS OF SHOES

We are drawn to certain colours when we purchase a new pair of shoes. Some psychologists suggest that colour can account for 60% of the acceptance or rejection of a product. In shoes it's probably higher.

Colours affect our psyches even when we are not consciously aware of them. Vision is not the only form of physiological reaction humans have to the colour spectrum. Preliminary scientific studies show that red radiation is more likely to produce epileptic seizures than blue. When blood pressure, respiration, heart rate, and the amount of times we blink, are measured, the colour red results in increasing the rate or frequency, while blue produces the lowest rate. Thus the cooler the colour, the more we can see it as having a calming effect. Painting your bedroom bright orange may be funky, but certainly not relaxing! It is paradoxical that the lower the frequency of the colour, the greater its ability to increase our heart rate. Just think of red and its association with prostitutes and the so-called red light districts! If we can accept this scientifically proven response to colour, then it is not hard to believe that our shoe colour selection is also affected by our mood.

Does colour have an effect on our emotions and behaviour? The answer is yes. But in terms of what kind of effect and how, the findings are inconclusive. Our reactions to colours are led by a combination of biological, physiological, psychological, social and cultural factors.

Throughout history, we have used fashion to differentiate ourselves, to state our uniqueness, our social class, our gender, even our age group. From the Yuppie in Armani suits, to the black clothing and body-piercing of Goth teenagers, to the dressed for success woman's business suit, clothing is a way of conveying our outward persona or rather how we would like to be seen.

Colours often have different symbolic meanings in different cultures. For example, white is the colour for weddings in the west, but in traditional Chinese culture white is worn for funerals. Red is known in the West as symbolizing anger and passion, while the Chinese associate it with happiness. In the West, the colour blue is associated with boys while little girls are made to wear pink, a concept not shared in the East.

Bearing in mind that different cultures may not view colours as having the same meaning, we can, through a western viewpoint, examine the choice of our shoes as relates to their colour and its ability to reflect our emotional states.

The most common shoe colours are brown and black. This is not surprising when we consider that what our shoes connect to is the earth, which is usually brown or dark brown/black. Wearing these colours indicates an earthiness or desire to ground ourselves and connect with the earth, while brighter more vibrant colours show a desire to elevate the self.

Black

KEY ISSUES
Feminine. Shadow. Intuition. Unknown. Death. Need to feel grounded.

Black can indicate someone who is mysterious, sexy and elusive. It can have dark or ominous connotations such as in black moods, depression, or having a dark personality. The image of a siren comes to mind. It can also referring to our shadow side - the aspects of our psyche that we keep hidden from others. Wearing black at funerals, indicates both the soul's departure into the unknown and our own withdrawal from society into our inner selves, as we come to terms with the loss. We can also *step into the unknown* or seduce others to do so. It may also be a desire to connect with the earth and the inner feminine self.

Blue

KEY ISSUES
Calm. Peace. Truth. Depressed.

Someone who is calm, peaceful, truthful and able to manifest what they need in their lives. If dirty, then it can indicate depression as in *feeling blue*.

Brown

KEY ISSUES
Earthy.

This person is practical, grounded and earthy; strongly rooted, so change could be difficult; someone who can be relied upon. If dirty, brown can indicate a withdrawn and introverted nature. It is not surprising that brown is the most popular colour in footwear if you include all ages and sexes. Besides its practical colouring being made from animal hide, on a symbolic level it is our attempt to remain grounded in our reality.

Gold

KEY ISSUES
Wealth, both financial and spiritual. Ruler.

As in silver it can indicate wealth or attachment to wealth. Also indicates a desire to rule (royalty wears gold) which could mean a desire to control and dominate others. It can also indicate supreme illumination as the reward for achieving a perfected state, as in the pot of gold at the end of the rainbow. The rainbow with its seven-coloured rays contains all aspects of us that need to be mastered to achieve this.

Green

KEY ISSUES
Healing. Growth. Balance. Envy.

A balanced and compassionate person who Gives and receives love. This could be a growth stage in your life. If dirty, you could be jealous of someone or something, as in *green with envy*.

Grey

KEY ISSUES
Lifeless. Dull. Exhaustion. Indecisive. Wisdom.

Are you uncertain about where you are going in life as in *grey areas*? Has life become dull and grey? Are you tired and feeling washed out? It can also denote wisdom, as in the graying of hair that together with wisdom, comes with old age. In old age we become emotionally withdrawn from the world around us.

Orange

KEY ISSUES
Happiness. Enthusiasm. Feeling. Fun. Warmth.
Orange is the colour of feeling and assimilation of feelings. In its purest state it indicates an emotionally uplifted state, as in the robes worn by Hindu yogis and swamis. It is a vibrant, social, warm and optimistic colour. It can also indicate carrying guilt if the orange is muddy. It can indicate one who serves others.

Pink

KEY ISSUES
Love. Compassion.

A loving person who is caring and compassionate. A dirty pink can indicate the need to draw strength from others in relationships.

Red

KEY ISSUES
Energy. Passion. Danger. Anger/aggression.

If your preferred choice of colour is red, then you are vibrant, energetic and passionate. It could also indicate anger and a fiery temper, as in *seeing red.*

Silver

KEY ISSUES
The moon/feminine. Mystical. Magical.

The moon is described as being silver. The moon is magical, mystical and feminine. It can also relate to wealth.

Purple
See Violet, but more intense.

Turquoise

KEY ISSUES
Self-expression. Manifestation.

This is the colour of self-expression and speaking one's truth. Good to wear if you need to give a lecture.

Violet

KEY ISSUES
Wisdom. Intuition. Inspiration.

Ruled by Venus, the Violet flower can represent enchantment or being charming, as well as spiritual wisdom as, other than white, it is the colour with the highest vibration.

White

KEY ISSUES
Purity. Clarity. Wholeness. Lightness.

Because all the colours of the spectrum are contained in white it represents wholeness. White has the highest rate of vibration. May be the colour of the perfectionist. Also indicates a desire for spiritual ascension.

Yellow

KEY ISSUES
Sun/male energy. Transformation. Mental abilities. Self-esteem. Cowardice.

Yellow can reflect a warm sunny person with good self-esteem; possibly an extrovert. Able to fight for what they believe is right and having good mental capabilities. This person embraces change. If the yellow is dirty, it can indicate cowardice, such as *yellow belly*.

Numbers of pairs of shoes

Do you have hoards of shoes, some of which you have barely worn? Is shoe collecting your thing? I once worked with a man who had over twenty pairs of Western boots in various styles. By wearing his boots (and Stetsons!) even though he was a born and bred South

African, he was making a statement of his desire to be seen as strong and masculine.

He was small fry compared to former Philippine First Lady, Mrs. Imelda Marcos. While her fellow countrymen lived in abject poverty, Mrs. Marcos is said to have owned over 1,500 pairs of shoes. She eventually opened her own museum, where most of the exhibits were her shoes.

Why do some people have have many, many of pairs of shoes? Perhaps they are trying to perform, or act out too many different roles in life, as in *filling too many shoes*. Perhaps they are unsure of what they want in life and so enjoy trying out different roles?

No shoes at all

If the shoes you wear is revealing, then what does being barefoot say about you? Many prophets, mystics and sages wandered through deserts and mountains barefoot, as a sign of humility. Our feet are incredible sensory organs; when they are kept in shoes they are seldom able to reveal their abilities.

Being barefoot is also a way to connect with the earth. Children, for the most part, particularly in hot countries, loathe shoes and remove them at the first opportunity. It is incredibly healthy to feel this connection to the ground, and at the same time receive a natural massage from the earth.

Squashed Toes

KEY ISSUES

Literally thoughts/beliefs/ideas crushed, pushed aside, stifled and suppressed. No space to bring ideas into reality or follow up on them. Dominated by other toes and what they represent. Abusive treatment.

PHYSICAL CAUSES

People with bunions often have squashed toes. As the bunion pushes outwards, the big toe turns inwards, squashing the adjacent toes. There are however, many other people who don't have bunions, but whose toes are squashed. Most common in the cases I have seen, is the second toe that squashes the third toe, with the result that the third toe is hardly visible from the top of the foot.

EMOTIONAL CAUSES

Squashed or smothered toes relate to our thoughts of being squashed. We may not have room to think. Or others may stifle or override our ideas and force us to conform to their way of thinking. If the **second toe** is squashed, a person may battle to establish a healthy sense of self-love. A partner may push their thoughts aside. It may also be that it is their own feelings and needs that they find hard to express. If the **third toe** is squashed, they may lack self-esteem and the ability to fight for what they believe is right. They may have lost their sense of self, in the constant need to please others, who frequently hammer down their ideas. This may result in a considerable amount of repressed aggression. If the **fourth toe** is squashed, they may have allowed their ideas to be trampled on by others; alternatively they may *bend over backwards* to adapt to others' ideas. If the **baby toe** is squashed, they may turn their backs on the beliefs that they were with, or later they may repress their own ideas in order to conform to the beliefs of their family.

CASE STUDY

Lara was a businesswoman in her late thirties. She managed a number of clothing retail outlets and was clearly financially successful. Coming to see me had been the result of a gift from a friend, who recognized Lara's need. She came from a large family of five siblings whose mother had died of cancer when Lara was only thirteen. She had assumed responsibility for the raising of her three younger siblings (her older brother and sister were already away at college). On meeting her I found it hard to believe this shy, withdrawn unconfident person held the position she did.

The second toe (heart chakra) on her right foot was hidden by the first and third toes. Squashed out to the back it was barely visible from the top of the foot. After explaining the significance of the left and right foot, I asked her if she felt that she was being dominated or smothered by her partner. How much did she feel that she was being nurtured by him and how much was he repressing her. She said she did not feel nurtured and she had closed her heart to a relationship that did not provide her with love or intimacy. Large calluses over her heart reflex on both feet also highlighted her need to protect herself. The calluses were yellow and so I asked if she was fed up about this. She replied that she was. The shininess on the callus also related to friction with her husband, which she could relate to.

She had a large bunion on her left foot. Realizing then that this did not relate to her past I asked her if there was someone who was very authoritative and critical of her. She replied that her husband was constantly finding fault with her, which didn't surprise me given the squashed second toe. Her relationship had crushed her. I suggested then that in order to counteract his criticism she perhaps pushed herself to win the approval, which he withheld. She agreed and we discussed how his manipulative behaviour could be controlling her. What was really behind the stress was the feeling that only by succeeding at work was she of any value. If she gave up her job, which she could afford to do, then she would have no value whatsoever. She would never be perfect in his view, because he could not accept his own imperfection or faults. Trying then to achieve his love was an impossible goal.

There was also a line up between her first three toes and the remaining big and heart/fourth toe on the left foot. I asked her if she felt divided in some way between two aspects of her life and she said she felt pulled between her spiritual growth and the work/pressure/ relationship with her hubby who was not prepared to change and was fearful of her exploring anything spiritual. Her feet were quite white in areas and this, together with her sunken adrenal reflexes, related to her exhaustion.

Crossing lines on the instep below the ball of the left foot suggested that she was not sure which direction to take. Lara agreed that this was so. Also under the second toe neck of the left foot there was a band of stretched skin almost choking the toe. I asked if she found it difficult to express her heartfelt emotions and she commented that she had found it easier to suppress (swallow) them which matched the feeling this toe neck gave me.

The small toes were separate from the other toes (more on the left) so I asked if she needed space from her family or colleagues, or if she felt removed from them. She said the first was true as with such a big family in the past and now with a demanding office situation in the present she needed space to think.

We spoke about her critical husband who saw her achievement as a threat. Resenting her success, which far surpassed his career achievements, he expressed his resentment by constantly criticizing her and making her feel not good enough. Hence, like the toe, she withdrew from him, sexually and emotionally. But she put huge pressure on herself to achieve, sacrificing what was really important to her such, as time with the children, friends and so on. She found it easier to escape into work, rather than dealing with her emotions and her relationship issues.

All of this she understood. While I was massaging her later, she said she felt as if huge weights were being lifted from her. When she left she said she felt much lighter and determined to work at resolving as opposed to avoiding her marital issues. She also planned to spend some time alone each day to connect with herself and her feelings.

HEALING

When one of your toes is squashed, it's time to examine your life, to look for where you are being squashed or restricted in some way, just like a plant that is squashed in amongst too many other plants has to fight to grow stronger and find the light. Who is dominating you? Do they have a right to? What is happening to your spirit as a result of this? What is more important, living fully and freely, or living safely? There is only one time. Now. Tomorrow may be too late. Carpe Diem! Work at freeing yourself from restrictions that you and others have placed upon yourself. If you don't it's unlikely anyone else will. Take a break and review your life. Give yourself space to think clearly about what kind of future you desire.

Splinters and Thorns

KEY ISSUES

Feeling invaded or intruded upon. Some external threat.

EMOTIONAL ISSUES

A splinter or thorn is an invasive element that causes us much pain. When you get a *thorn in your flesh,* you need to ask yourself what is causing you so much discomfort or hurt. Is it a *thorny* situation or is someone in particular a *thorn in your side?* Thorns and splinters pierce our flesh unexpectedly, so there could be an aspect of surprise or an unexpected revelation about a situation. The larger the thorn or splinter, the greater the pain and the bigger the emotional situation is likely to be.

ORIGIN OF WORD

Splinter derives from the word split. Being pierced by a splinter then also has origins in being split or cut-up.

CASE STUDY

Case one: A client had a two cm splinter pierce through the heart chakra on her left foot. It had occurred quite suddenly stepping off a jetty while on holiday. The splinter was so deep that surgery was required to remove it and several stitches needed. The poor woman was on crutches for weeks after. Clearly something had *pierced her flesh* and was making her very *heartsore.* The situation kept her bedridden for several days, during which time she was forced to slow down and reflect on her life in general and the situation that was causing her so much pain.

Chatting about her life she realized that she had indeed reached some sort of *heartfelt* crisis in her life which needed urgent examination. Her *heart was torn* between the security of a job she had held as a psychologist in the same position for the past twenty years and the obligation she felt to her family versus her own desire to explore herself and expand her potential. She admitted feeling cut-up about the situation.

Case two: A petite woman in her early thirties suffered a similar invasion, although for different reasons. The two cm splinter that pierced the upper instep (third chakra) area, in line with the third toe on the right foot went so deep that surgery was also required to remove it. The wound then went septic and only speedy medical intervention stopped the spread of gangrene.

This invasive splinter pierced her spleen chakra, which has to do with expressing anger or *venting ones spleen*. Being in the third chakra area and below the third toe, it also had to do with feeling that her self-esteem and her confidence had been wounded. Because the damage was on the right foot it naturally involved a man and also had to do with a past, unresolved issue that had recently been brought to a head. Realizing the full extent of just how toxic the relationship had been (he had been unfaithful throughout their marriage), was very emotionally disturbing and wounded her deeply.

The subsequent serious infection, in spite of having had early medical intervention, mirrored the emotional poison that the situation had spewed forth. The resulting foul smell from the infection, showed just how unpleasant and putrid the whole situation had become. Realizing this she was able to get rid not only of the morbid and putrid thoughts regarding him, but physically she was able to cut him out of her life.

HEALING:

Identify who or what the *thorn in your side* might be and work at emotionally removing or rectifying the situation. In making certain the wound is clean, you ensure that you have cleaned away the problem. Depending on the size of the thorn, this could be a serious wake-up call and a prod to change something in your life, or address an issue.

Sweaty/Smelly Feet

KEY ISSUES

Fear. Worry, often over small matters.

PHYSICAL CAUSES

If you wear synthetic trainers (running shoes), particularly without socks, after a few weeks only the dog will find them desirable, even if they did cost the greater part of your disposable income. We all sweat as it is essential to maintaining healthy bodily functions. As we sweat the moisture evaporates, cooling our bodies down. We also excrete harmful toxins and regulate the balance of salt in our systems. Fiery foods, such as curry, alcohol, hot spices as well as smoking, drinking coffee and fevers increase the amount we sweat. The sweat glands are controlled by the nervous system. Stale sweat carries a bad odour, so smelly shoes are very common. However, there are certain people, whose less than fragrant feet become legend in their environment. They clearly sweat more and there is an emotional reason for this.

EMOTIONAL CAUSES

You've heard about those people who *sweat the small stuff*? and who allow the smallest of problems to create a huge amount of concern. Because sweating is controlled by the nervous system, excessive sweating may be an indication that we are by nature afraid or nervous. Often we are in a flight or fight situation And we drink alcohol or coffee and smoke as ways to try to calm ourselves down, or create a *smokescreen* between us and what we fear. Eating fiery foods is a way to build up our fire or warrior energy, when we may be feeling watery or carry too much of the feminine principle. Excessive sweating excretes what we have been feeling insecure about. When stale as a result of fear or aggression, sweat has a distinctive odor. Do you find yourself in a situation that *stinks*? If we constantly sweat, it may be an indication that we are living in fear.

Excessive sweating usually mirrors emotions that have been bottled up. Anger is not the only cause and may simply be a mask for deeper feelings of fear or shame. A burning sensation in the feet can result, which shows that we are literally fuming inside. When excessive smell is involved, the situation may have reached the point that it literally stinks!

ORIGIN OF WORD

The word smell originates from *smolen*, which means to smoulder. Smouldering indicates a suppressed anger than burns within us. Often the real anger/fear/sadness may be with ourselves, although we may project that onto another person.

CASE STUDY

I recall being told by a mother about how she had had her son's sweat glands removed in both the hands and feet, as he sweated profusely. As this is a reasonably serious operation involving a full anesthetic, it seemed a fairly drastic move. Perhaps, instead of immediately turning to invasive surgery, it would have been less traumatic for the child, at least as a first step, to examine whether there were fear issues involved, particularly as the boy was very sensitive. The sweating situation was worse during tests and exams, so clearly the child had a fear of not performing well. Maybe examining why the child was so afraid of failure, and then dealing with it might have gone a long way toward alleviating the situation.

HEALING

We need to find ways to express what we suppress. Art, writing a journal, therapy, sport all may assist the process. We also need to work with trust and security issues and accept the underlying situation that we are afraid of and then release the anger on the surface. This boy in the above situation, may have been really afraid of not achieving well and meeting his parent's expectations. Trying to comply with their desires against his own, may have caused a deep-rooted anger, which he was afraid to express. The stink his feet caused, was a subconscious expression of the desire he had to *cause a stink*.

Swollen Feet

KEY ISSUES

Repressed emotions.

PHYSICAL CAUSES

Swelling may be caused by an obstruction in the lymphatic system, or as a result of injury or infection. The swelling is the body's attempt to repair the damage or fight the infection, as surrounding blood vessels open up and send an increased amount of oxygen, nutrition and white blood cells into the area.

EMOTIONAL CAUSES

When a part of our feet, or toes are swollen, it is an indication that we have a large build-up of emotion. We have contained an issue for so long that it threatens to burst our emotional selves.

CASE STUDY

An elderly client had a very swollen fourth toe on her right foot (past issues), and a less swollen second toe on her left foot. Although not painful, they had caused the underlying area in the heart area to be sore. She mentioned that she had had these swollen toes for many years. I asked whether she might be holding onto or unable to express an issue to do with guilt (second chakra) that might have affected a past relationship and that had possibly made her heartsore.

She then told me a very moving story about her childhood. She had a sister, two years younger than herself and towards whom she had felt a huge amount of resentment. Sibling rivalry was intensified by the remoteness of their home, a father who had little time for his daughters and a sick mother. Life had not been easy as her mother had suffered from depression and had little energy to give her daughters as the nature of depression is that we are depleted of energy. Thus the little there was in the way of love was fought over by the sisters, with the younger, cuter sister inevitably winning.

One day while playing with her sister, the younger child had taken my client's favorite doll and pulled its hair out. My client was so enraged at the destruction that she had yelled out, "I wish you were dead!" Under the circumstances, this was a perfectly understandable response from an eight-year old child. However, her younger sister contracted an illness shortly after this incident and died two weeks later. As children are inclined to do, my client assumed responsibility for her sister's death and had been too afraid to reveal to any adult the burden of guilt she carried. Now, more than sixty years later, her swollen toes revealed that she still carried a huge amount of guilt, although as an adult she was aware that she was not to blame. Linking the swollen toes with her sister's death brought a depth of understanding to the issue and we suggested ways that she could work at and come to terms with forgiving her own inner child.

HEALING

Whenever there is something swollen, it is an indication of an emotion that needs to be released. We need to examine where the swelling is in order to be able to determine what type of emotion has caused this build-up of feeling. For instance, guilt will lie in the second chakra, anger in the third etc. Finding a way to express this emotion will relieve the pressure.

Toe Length

KEY ISSUES

Creative potential. Leadership abilities. Unique ideas. Possible arrogance.

PHYSICAL CAUSES

Morton's Toe, where the second toe is longer than the big toe, is a common occurrence. On some people though it can lead to excessive pressure and pain being exerted on the bone at its base on the ball of the foot.

EMOTIONAL CAUSES

The longer your toes, the longer your 'antennae,' and therefore the greater your potential for receiving thoughts and ideas from the universe and finding ways to them 'out there.' People with long toes are more likely to think creatively, while very short-toed people may be better at implementing these ideas. Often their long-toed buddies may have their heads up in the clouds seeking more ideas and yet are unable to cope with the practical detail implementing these ideas entail.

When toes are bent, it is a sign that our creative potential has been pushed back, either by others or our own fear of shouldering not only the responsibility of our creation, but its potential failure as well. We may also be so airy, that we battle to *get a grip on* reality, as in the case of the absent minded professor. Our toes try to grip onto earthly reality to stop us floating off in some etheric conceptual direction.

In the film *Shallow Hal*, Hal's friend recounts having ended a relationship with an attractive girl because her second toe was longer than her big toe. Whether the knowledge was coincidental on the part of the scriptwriter or not, Hal's pal had a point, for a long second toe also relates to leadership potential, not at all the sort of woman Hal or his pal wanted!

CASE STUDY

Creativity should not be seen simply as being able to paint. Rather creativity can be found in practically every profession. A surgeon may be required to think very creatively about a better way to perform an operation; a journalist may need to create a whole different perspective when investigating an issue, and so on. I made the mistake of seeing creativity in too narrow a sphere in this next case.

A man in his early thirties came to see me. He had extremely long toes and I asked the question as to whether he had ever explored his creativity. He replied that he was not at all creative, being in the accounting world. Yet his toes were still long and not at all bent. I was confused. Surely he MUST be creative. Further discussion followed where he revealed that he was highly skilled at creating money with his various innovative schemes – there are very few men of his age who, through their own skills, do not HAVE to work. He had retired for a while to work with some new ideas he'd had. There seemed to be no pressing need to return to salaried employment. He knew that, when it became necessary, an idea would emerge and, when put into action, would provide him with even more wealth. He could not appreciate why other people found doing that so hard!

He also had a very large big toe, indicating his huge potential for the fifth chakra archetype of the alchemist or magician – he literally could turn base metal into gold and so in this way was extremely creative. He agreed with this and said it explained the relative ease he had in accumulating wealth.

HEALING

No matter what size or length your toes are, there is always potential for each and every one of us to access ideas and concepts and be creative. Having an innate ability is one thing, using it is quite another and many the tortoise that has surpassed the hare.

Varicose Veins

KEY ISSUES
Fear of standing up for oneself. Resentment. Feeling stuck. Feeling unsupported/burdened.

PHYSICAL CAUSES:
It's easy to understand how blood flows down through the legs to the feet as a result of gravity, but when it has to flow upwards, it requires small valves in the blood vessels which allow the blood to go up but not down. Should a few valves become faulty, then the flow of blood upwards becomes impeded, and the blood collects in the blood vessels which swell, causing prominent blue veins or varicose veins. Sometimes the swollen skin over the vein becomes irritated and the sufferer may well be driven to scratching, which can result in a type of eczema. Because of the slower blood flow, wounds can take longer to heal and may result in ulcers on the legs or feet. In some cases, the sluggish blood movement causes blood clots, which can move and block arteries in other parts of the body.

EMOTIONAL CAUSES
The blueness of the veins is an indication that the person concerned is feeling battered and bruised. Blaming long hours of standing on one's feet may be an indication that the person concerned is battling to stand up for themselves – the valves and weakened connective tissue are unable to push the blood higher up the body and the blood (our life force) settles in our lowest chakra. This relates to difficulties and, by extension, to a lethargic approach to moving ahead. When veins show up on the back of the foot, this indicates that we are dealing with issues from the past (or ones we felt were behind us), or issues that are subconscious and hidden from others.

When the swollen veins occur in pregnancy, we may be finding it hard to accept the new turn our lives are about to take. We may feel that the new baby will put even more of a burden on us and create more work than we can cope with, which naturally we might resent.

We may feel that others are not supporting us and, like our veins we simply want to collapse under the pressure of life. Our thinking, like our blood, may have become sluggish and we struggle to change preconceived ideas about the situation we find ourselves in. We may feel stuck in a situation we dislike, but can see no way to get out of it. If ulcers appear, the situation may have worsened to the point where we feel it is eating up our life force. If eczema develops and flares up in red, angry, sore patches (and particularly if it weeps) we are showing how intensely irritated we are with the situation, while the weeping mirrors the tears we have held back.

If wounds take longer to heal because the veins swell, this can reflect that we take longer to heal our emotional wounds or, in the case of swelling, that the hurt swells angrily inside us. Should the blood clot, instead of flowing freely, this shows us that our lives have become stagnant and not free or open to change.

CASE STUDY

Case one: Eve was a beautiful, fifty-something woman who ran a home industry. She had an aura of serene calmness about her and I warmed to her immediately. So it was a surprise when I saw that the tops of her feet were a myriad of varicose veins; somehow her feet did not seem to mirror the calmness she projected. In the many wonderful sessions we had together, her story began to unravel and I was able to understand both sides of Eve.

Eve had married very young, to a man many years older than herself. Together they had built up a profitable home industry, the responsibility of which, over the years, had fallen very much more on her shoulders. It was not a job that she was particularly interested in yet she had continued to perform her dutiful role, as the profit, according to her husband was worth the inconvenience. He had had a tough childhood and although he was in no way physically abusive to his family, as his father had been to him, he still controlled the family with a rod of verbal iron. There was only one way to do things – his way, and he rarely asked for input from his wife when it came to decision making. Forced into a career role that she did not enjoy, with little hope of changing things, she had learnt over the years to avoid challenging the status quo, telling herself philosophically that she must simply accept things as they were.

As we chatted, all the elements of varicose veins became clear: - her feelings and her fear of speaking out were stuck inside her, together with the belief that to ask for what she wanted was somehow being too demanding and not the spiritually correct thing to do. The pressure from the business left her feeling pressurized and burdened and she received little or no support from her husband. As the years went by she attempted to find her own identity, but her attempts were frequently met with undermining comments, until she almost felt it was wrong to have any desires outside the life she had. This inevitably led to her feeling resentment, which she suppressed. She hated where she was, yet saw little hope of ever being able to truly live her own life. She felt guilty for wanting more and resentful because she could not explore her world further without running into critical comment.

It was not difficult then to understand why she had developed an ulcer on the area of her uterus and vagina on the foot. The uterus, representing the area of creativity, was being eaten away by her sadness, frustration and anger at not being allowed to be a co-creator in her world.

Years of having her thoughts and feelings dominated had created the angry bruised appearance of her feet. However, as she began to hear her own inner voice, she learned to stand up for herself and start making claims for her right to live her life in a way that was appropriate to her. When last I heard from her, she had decided to take some time out – a kind of sabbatical – to reassess her life and search for what it was that she really wanted.

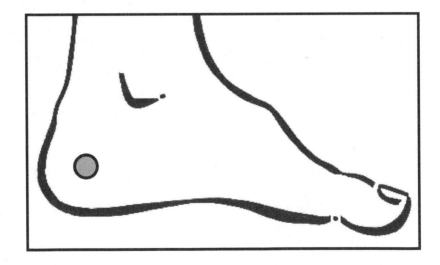

Fig. 44 · Ulcer on vagina area

Case Two: This was a case a friend reported to me, so I actually never met the people concerned; however, it was so interesting, that I have chosen to briefly describe it. Two elderly sisters were both found to have small varicose veins over the vagina area of their feet *(see Fig. 44)*. Further questioning revealed that both sisters had been raped when they were in their early twenties by different people, on different occasions; neither had ever told the other, or anyone else, at the time the rapes occurred, nor in the following years. (This was a pity because they could have provided a great deal of comfort to each other.) Both of them, understandably, carried resentment towards their rapists and both were still stuck in the wounds of the past, including resisting standing up to the perpetrators. Consequently they felt burdened by the secrets they had each carried for many years and this manifested in the visible veins on the area associated with the vagina on their feet.

PHYSICAL HEALING
Raising the legs to reverse the effects of gravity is a common way of gaining relief from varicose veins. In some cases support stockings may be recommended. In the long-term your medical practitioner may recommend the surgical removal of the veins concerned and /or injections into the smaller veins. Other veins then take over the function of those removed.

EMOTIONAL HEALING
Varicose veins occuring on the tops of the feet, relate to the back. This is where we hide things from others or where issues occur that we thought we had left behind. They can also relate to subconscious thoughts. Healing then involves identifying where we have stagnated; where we feel unsupported; and who or what is burdening us. Change is involved. We need to stand up for ourselves, release our resentment and move ahead with our lives, even if others do not approve of our actions. We are never truly stuck – stuckness is an illusion which we need to get rid of, if we are to find contentment. We need to take action or confront the situation, remove ourselves from it or surrender in acceptance to it if we want to release the emotional baggage we have invested in the situation.

Warts

KEY ISSUES
Feeling invaded. Expressions of hatred or dislike. Eaten up with repulsion.

PHYSICAL CAUSES
Warts are caused by a virus, which commonly invades the skin through very small cuts or abrasions. Technically, only those on the sole of the foot are referred to as Plantar warts, which are more prone to develop in children than in adults. In most cases, the warts are harmless, although they may cause pain, especially if they are on the load-bearing parts of the foot, such as the heel or ball. Warts, too, are sometimes mistaken for corns. In a few cases, more serious malignant lesions can also be thought to be warts and although rare, if one is concerned, it would be wise to consult a podiatric physician to get a diagnosis.

Plantar warts are raised areas that vary in colour from grey to brown. The centre appears as a few pinpoints of black. Plantar warts can be very resistant to treatment. I have tried numerous allopathic, homeopathic and herbal remedies with only varying degrees of success, when they developed on the foot of one of my children. Having got rid of them once, they can reoccur.

Like Athlete's Foot they are said to be contracted from walking on dirty surfaces or in warm, moist environments such as gyms and swimming pools. If untreated they can grow and multiply, as the host inadvertently touches and spreads the virus. If scratched, the resulting blood can also be a carrier for the virus. That being said, when my daughter had warts, in spite of our communal bathroom facilities, none of us caught the virus.

EMOTIONAL CAUSES
The fact that viruses are external organisms that invade us is a big clue to their origin. When we have a wart, we are literally being invaded in some aspect of our lives. We feel incapable of expelling this unwanted intruder. As the warts break through our skin, boundary issues are involved. We might want to stand up against the issue or person, but feel incapable of doing so. The pain a wart can cause is also an indication of how painful a particular situation can be.

Witches were commonly depicted with warts and frogs or toads have been thought to carry the fungus. Both outcasts and considered undesirable and unlovable, the horny toad and the ugly witch may hint of aspects of ourselves that we find repulsive or unacceptable. Both have been associated mythically with ugliness and the darker, shadow aspects of ourselves. So it may be that it is dark, *ugly* thoughts that invade us, rather than something external. Depending on where on the foot they are found, that would indicate what specific aspects of ourselves we dislike. Accepting someone *warts and all*, is to accept them, in spite of their deficiencies.

Children often feel unprotected against the invasion of their space by siblings. They may harbor deep and dark thoughts about those who compete for their parent's attention while at the same time loving them. When we have warts, the person whom we are having the problem with is usually someone within the household.

Warts on the ball of the foot: the soft fleshy ball of the foot relates to the heart and lungs (heart/fourth chakra). Warts on this area then could indicate small expressions of self-hatred, feeling unlovable, and ashamed of ourselves, which then could make it hard to accept ourselves. Or, it may be someone else who is emotionally invading our heart space and whom we feel powerless to stand up to.

CASE STUDY

Case one: I had a client whose heart reflex mirrored very graphically her traumatic relationship. Rebecca was a beautifully ethereal person, who told me she worked as a holistic healer. After the initial examination, I noticed a wart on her right foot's heart area. Warts as you know, have to do with feeling invaded and this invasion, particularly in the area of our hearts, causes dislike, even revulsion, at something we seem powerless to stop. The roots of this invasion penetrate our core and destroy any boundaries we may have created.

I asked if she was presently experiencing a relationship that felt invasive and which may be causing her to dislike or be repelled by someone else's actions. She said she had experienced deep grief and anguish when a lover had consciously infected her with a Sexually Transmitted Disease (STD). She was very angry with him and revolted, not just by the STD, but with herself for having entered into a liaison that she knew was invasive and had broken all her boundaries. Yellow calluses over the whole heart area, also showed her resentment and vulnerability. In addition to having calluses, the underside of the heart area of the foot was very flat, as if all joyful emotion had been drained from her. (This may also have had to do with having nurtured her clients to the point of feeling drained herself.)

When I enquired a week later as to how she was, she said the callus over her heart (area) had peeled off and the wart was in the process of coming away. She felt this was an indication that this whole part of her life had shifted and she could now leave it where it belonged – in the past.

Case two: Jessica was a pretty ten-year old girl, tall for her age, and clearly intelligent, although her school marks did not reflect this, as she had a learning difficulty. She was, her mother told me, a loner who struggled to be included in social activities with her peers. Much of the time she sat alone at break-time and although she had had two close friends in the past, both had left the school. She rarely invited friends to her home and instead spent much of her time alone, playing with her pets or day-dreaming.

The only major upset in her life had been the birth of her baby brother, which affected her deeply. As she was very close to her mother, the four years that separated the siblings was enough to ensure that the new arrival brought Jessica huge emotional upheaval and she obviously saw her brother as an intruder into her relationship with her mother. The new arrival was a difficult baby who demanded much of her mother's time and attention and Jessica was forced to assume a lesser role in the family, in spite of efforts to the contrary. She went from being a happy, enthusiastic and outgoing child to a quiet, withdrawn loner. As the baby grew up, he became quite physically abusive to his older sister, who stoically accepted the pinches and thumps (although occasionally she did surreptitiously pinch her brother back). As much as her brother was 'bad,' to those who had not witnessed her odd acts of aggression, Jessica was angelic.

Now, six years later, she had developed four warts on her right foot.

The first was on the third toe on the lower part of the toe pad. Sibling rivalry had become a big aspect of her life. As I've mentioned before, noses have to do with the need for recognition and Jessica's nose was *out of joint* as she felt her brother's achievements outshone hers and she was not getting the recognition from her parents she yearned for. The warts represented small expressions of hatred she felt towards both her sibling (and her mother) whom she felt had betrayed her by having another child. She felt her brother, who had caused a complete upheaval in her life, had invaded her home. The warts also symbolized the 'intruder' eating into her self-esteem.

A second wart on the heart or the neck of the second toe showed that she had problems expressing this anger; instead it festered inside. How could she who had assumed the role of a good sweet child, express vile and unpleasant feelings, particularly towards someone her parents loved?

Another wart was on the center of the toe pad on this same toe. Being on the second/heart toe had to do with her one-on-one relationships and how she saw them. She felt her brother had taken away much of the joy she had experienced before his birth and the situation eroded her self-esteem, making her unsure of who she was. She wasn't sure how to react or who to turn to, as her father was a busy man and had little time to share with her.

The fourth wart was very large and below the ball of the foot, in the area of the solar plexus. Our solar plexus is in the third chakra and has to do with self-esteem and the ability to fight for what we believe is right. It also has to do with anger. Jessica clearly had problems expressing her anger and she had adopted the role of 'angel' in opposition to her tyrannical brother. As angels don't hit, bite, throw temper tantrums and pinch, she had no natural way to express her pent-up resentment. Instead it bottled up inside her, appearing as warts, which broke through the strong, controlled walls she had created around herself.

As I looked at her feet, I was filled with sadness for her. Other relevant features included her heart reflex on the same foot, which was covered in hardened skin, indicating how she had felt the need to protect herself from feeling vulnerable or exposing herself to verbal or emotional attack. The thymus also had a wall of protection on this foot only, showing her need to protect her time and space. This was reflected in her need to be alone. Shortly before coming to see me, she had also cut open her right foot, on the shoulder area, which had required stitches.

Shouldering this burden of anger and vile thoughts and yet feeling guilty for having so much hatred towards her brother had *cut her up*. A line on her heart chakra on this foot also indicated that the birth of her brother had broken her heart. Jessica also often had bad breath, symbolizing the festering of vile and angry feelings she was unable to express.

As I talked with Jessica about her feelings towards her sibling, she gradually opened up and shared the secret thoughts she harbored. Her mother too, once she understood the full depth of the child's angst was able to create special times when just the two of them could do activities alone. It took a long time, but eventually the warts fell off on their own. As the skin peeled away this reflected a new growth in the relationship between Jessica and her mother and behaviour between the siblings became more natural with a fair amount of physical interplay on both sides. Taking up judo also helped give Jessica a valid outlet for her aggression. Realizing that his older sister would now retaliate, the younger boy stopped his attacks and harmony was restored. The warts had not returned in the following two years and hopefully never will.

PHYSICAL HEALING

Having warts professionally removed either involves a wart removal preparation or in extreme cases a simple surgical procedure under local anaesthetic. Sometimes they are frozen off with liquid nitrogen. Laser removal is also common. Over the counter treatments can damage the healthy surrounding skin and must be applied with care.

EMOTIONAL HEALING

Do you feel invaded? Is someone penetrating your space leaving you feeling vulnerable? Are you battling to accept yourself *warts and all*? What do you feel ashamed about? Where do you hold guilt? Do you find aspects of yourself ugly and try to separate yourself from them? "What has got into you?" is something we often hear mothers say to their children. What then that you view as unpleasant, has become part of you? Answers to these questions may help to understand why you have developed warts.

Wrinkles and Lines

KEY ISSUES
Represents barriers. Conflicting issues. Changing directions/thinking.

EMOTIONAL ISSUES
Walking on flat ground is far easier than hiking up and down hills And so, on our feet the, 'hills' or wrinkles represent the ups and downs that we have had, or are currently experiencing in life – and it's not surprising then that they are so common in the area representing relationships and our relationship to ourselves! All these extra hills complicate our lives and drain our energy, so ask yourself "Is this hill worth all the time and energy it takes to climb?" next time you encounter an issue that exhausts you.

We often find large ripples on the second chakra of our feet, indicating the difficulty we have with relationships, money, sexuality, and the accompanying guilt we feel. The presence of these wrinkles represents the challenges of life, as opposed to having a smooth ride (no wrinkles). Women very often carry so much guilt, particularly an area that relates to our children. Also if we feel we can't move on and leave our emotional stuff behind, our feet may become wrinkled in this area to reflect the rut we are stuck in.

Lines drawn across a page divide one part from another and the same can be said about the lines on our feet. We may either want to separate aspects of our lives, or perhaps we feel divided on an issue. These lines can also draw attention to, and thus a way of accessing an issue. Lines represent impediments, obstacles or blockages that stifle our ability to move and, if on the throat (neck of the toes) they are like a cord that strangles our ability to speak our truth. If we have deep vertical lines across the second chakra, they indicate difficulties in relationships that have to be overcome. On the third chakra, horizontal lines can indicate difficulties we have to overcome in relation to our self-esteem and relationship to self. A distinct line between the fourth and third toe shows a need to separate our heart and emotions from our sense of self. We don't want to feel our feelings, as they threaten us, so we create a divide or cut them off.

Sometimes lines can create certain images, such as a net to indicate that we feel trapped, or a funnel to show where we are being drained. Scattered lines may indicate we feel scattered, while "V" shaped lines

189

may show we do not know which path to follow. A line across the heart reflex shows we have suffered a broken heart.

CASE STUDY

Case One: Line across heart: It always saddens me to see the number of people who have lines across their heart area. One of many cases I have seen of these lines was exemplified by Claire, a middle-aged woman, who had immigrated with her husband and family back to Scotland, the country of her birth. One disaster followed another and they finally packed it in and returned to Australia, her husband's birth place. She was deeply saddened by this, together with the financial loss they faced. She was angry with her husband for not having succeeded in Scotland and very divided now between her love for her country and having to accept that she would most likely never live there again. The deep dividing and calloused line over the heart chakra between the big and second toes indicated the divide she felt from having to live in one country while wanting to be in another.

Claire could relate to having a broken heart; her life had simply become completely different from the way she had planned and she was almost in shock at the way her life had turned out. Interestingly, she also had deep, net-like lines on her feet. As mentioned above, a net indicates we feel trapped and Claire could relate well to the net representing her feelings about being stuck in a country where she didn't want to be, with a man she resented. While there seemed to be no solution to her problem, having shared her feelings and having them acknowledged, did help to ease her pain.

Case Two: Line between solar plexus and heart chakra. When there is no joy in our lives, it is as if our life-force has been drained. We lack enthusiasm (which comes from the Greek *enthous* meaning "possessed by God") and we feel we have little God or Divine energy in our lives; and rather than our higher selves prevailing our negative ego rules supreme. Thus all we can see is negativity, hopelessness, separation, failure and lack. We have become separated from the Divine; we have *burnt* ourselves *out*; our fire or energy is depleted; and our watery passivity now puts us out of balance. The feet become flaccid and when the skin on the sole is pressed it takes a while to push itself back. The feet are white or drained of colour, showing how exhausted we are. The adrenal glands are sunken showing that we have been living in a fight or flight mentality for a long time.

Kim's feet were as described above, plus she had a deep line just above the solar plexus on both feet showing how she had become detached from her heart or emotions. There were also numerous other ridges on her insteps. There was also a large callused line on her heart chakra between the big and second toes that reached down to the third chakra, meaning that her divide had an impact on her energy. The situation had become so bad in Kim's case, that she had developed Chronic Fatigue Immune Deficiency, also known as ME. Driven by a desire to achieve, to compensate for her fear of failure and feelings of inadequacy, Kim had worked long and hard in maintaining her clients in her interior design business.

But ME is more than just physical exhaustion, it is about a spiritual inner conflict between our higher and lower selves. When we avoid following our spiritual needs, we often fall into the victim trap where our ego is in control. We become obsessed with our physical and emotional selves to compensate for a lack of connection to our spiritual selves. Life can become all about **ME**, **my** illness, **my** needs, and **my** issues. Like the ego we also see ourselves as being "special." We can become very needy for attention, yet our ego prevents us from asking for it.

In this case Kim's dividing line could be said to represent the divide between her higher and ego selves. The very thick calluses on both pituitary glands, and the big toes turned sharply inwards, indicated how she had blocked off her spirituality. She was too afraid to explore this, for fear of not being in control or "succeeding." As in the case of Adam and Eve we have become separated from what has real meaning in our lives. Our lives are battles to fight the giant monster that is our ego. Like the mythic knight we need to slay the powerful ego dragon. Not engaging this path had left Kim without purpose. Life had become too hard to be a part of,it was easier to give-up rather than go on as accepting the challenge would take huge courage and commitment Perhaps, as she was in the process of selling her business and had initiated coming to have Reiki and a foot treatment, this was an indication that she has was just beginning to take up that challenge.

Case three: Line across colon. Natasha had a very deep line on the lower instep of her left foot and also one on the heel over the area of the colon; although there was also a line her right foot, it was more pronounced on the left. It was so deep it looked like a cut and I asked her if she had had an accident. When she replied she hadn't, my next question was about surgery. Indeed, three months prior to her visit to me, Natasha had undergone surgery for removal of part of her colon due to cancer. She said it had been about the time of the surgery that the lines had appeared on her foot and she had often wondered what had caused them. Now she had the answer.

She also had a deep line under her heart and above the solar plexus, as in the previous examples. When asked about the nature of the relationship with her partner, she revealed that things had been very unhappy for some time and they had talked of a divorce. Natasha felt that part of her colon trouble was related to issues about the relationship that she had held onto. She had been unable to digest and release the resentment and hurt this man had caused her. If she was to heal completely, Natasha would need to find some way to work through her emotions.

HEALING

In order to be whole (holy) we need to be integrated. Where we have lines is an indication, broadly speaking, that there are areas where we do not feel "together." We need then to ask what we have become separated from? Where do we feel divided? Do we lead a double life? Do we cut our head off from our hearts? Are we still cut-up for example, following a divorce? By addressing these issues we can start the process of healing the divide. If the lines resemble a net, ask yourself if you feel trapped and how you can free yourself.

Webbed Toes

KEY ISSUES

Deep connection between what is represented by the two toes that are webbed. If the second and the third toes are webbed, this would indicate that the person's ideas, heart-related issues and sense of self are more closely linked. They would act from the heart.

PHYSICAL CAUSES

If you draw an imaginary line between the base of the neck of the small toe and the base of the big toe, the toes normally line up along that line. Where one or more join higher up, they can be said to be webbed and most often it occurs between the second and third toes. The toes (and fingers) are connected by a small piece of tissue, either all the way to the ends of the digits or just at the base. The connection consists of just skin and soft tissue. Separating the toes if cosmetically required is relatively easy, although care must be taken not to sever the arteries going to each toe.

EMOTIONAL CAUSES

One of the 32 signs that indicated the Buddha's greatness and future role as redeemer and spiritual ruler was webbed fingers and toes. His toes were reported to be long, his soles tender and soft, and his heels broad. (In reading his feet this would relate to being well grounded, being open to change, being flexible and having enormous potential.) Certain older statues of the Buddha, can be seen to have slight webbed fingers and toes.

It is reported that more children are being born now with webbed toes, a feature which is particularly linked to "Indigo children." These children seem to have great spiritual depth and often have gifts such as physic powers. Much has been written about them in recent years. They are not necessarily easy to raise as they have very strong wills, they may also be diagnosed as having Attention Deficit Hyperactivity Disorder (ADHD), and may also be mature beyond their years, they are an acknowledged phenomena. Most of these children (also known as Crystal children) have at least the third and fourth toes webbed and in some cases the second as well.

So what is the significance? Where two toes appear to be coming together as one, it mirrors that the attributes related to each toe are becoming more integrated. Thus, if the third and fourth toe were webbed, this would indicate a much closer relationship between you and your heart, particularly in your expression of love and your ideas regarding it. Heart and self are interdependent, and when this is truly so, you or your children are compassionate, loving, empathetic, creative, intelligent, intuitive, peaceful and well-balanced. Self-worth is not a big issue, you just know who you are and are okay with that. You are also able to express your needs; you are compassionate and have strong empathy for others; you are able to think abstractly and visualize well. Indeed, you display spiritual intelligence and wisdom beyond your years.

If the heart and the self are not interdependent then you would be more likely to have poor boundaries, be demanding, needy, may lack compassion for yourself and others and often feel isolated. You may feel "special" or superior to others, sometimes coming across as cold and callous; you may have difficulty conforming to discipline, authority and rules; you may feel a loner, isolated from your peers and misunderstood; you may refuse to do certain tasks and struggle to think beyond your immediate needs; and you may be emotionally (and sometimes physically) sensitive, or fragile, or distant.

And, like many people there can be times when you swing from balance to imbalance, sometimes feeling dependent and at other times feeling independent. Although Indigo children have been around for a long time, 1992 was the year attributed to greater numbers of such children being born. If your child was born after 1992 and has webbed toes, there's a very good chance he or she is an Indigo child. The following is an example of an 'older' Indigo child.

CASE STUDY

Annette had webbing on both feet between the second, third and fourth toes, which would indicate that she was an Indigo child (even though she was now in her sixties.) Related to the webbing, were the calluses found on both the pineal and pituitary glands. This indicated that she had closed the door on her spirituality and self-actualization. She had the potential to advance spiritually, but in discussions with her she revealed that she had shut the door on this aspect of her life, after being ridiculed for her abilities as a child. She had felt misunderstood and isolated and rather than continuing to feel this way, she had shut down her psychic potential in order to conform. It had simply been too painful, with strictly authoritarian, "stiff-upper-lip" parents to express any other behaviour. She said had displayed many of the positive aspects listed above. Like many highly sensitive and intuitive children, she had been misunderstood and her gift had been classified as curse. She had, therefore, repressed this aspect of herself, and turned away from her spiritual thoughts and ideas in order to conform to the familial culture, as the calluses showed. As her big toes (turning inwards) indicated, she now displayed some (although not all) of the more negative aspects of the heart and self split.

She had a huge heart area, which seemed to want to burst out at me. When we discussed her past and her potential for love, she became very tearful and felt that for the first time in her life she was being "seen" for who she really was. She said people with problems often came to her for a shoulder to cry on and she felt a deep sense of compassion and empathy for others, yet was hard on herself.

After she left, Annette emailed me to tell me she suddenly felt much "lighter," and in fact she lost a large amount of weight effortlessly shortly thereafter.

HEALING

Simply acknowledging that you are equipped with the ability to feel more and have great compassion, may be all that needs to occur for you to accept your role in life. Knowing that you have closer communication between various aspects of yourself may help you to understand those who do not. Webbed feet are a mark of huge potential – use it!

Endnotes

Introduction

1 Hermes Trismegistos, *The Emerald Tablet* (translated by Adept Ful-canelli) as quoted in *Alchemists and Gold: The Story of Alchemy Through the Ages* by Jaques Sadoul (New York: G.P. Putnam, 1972).

2 Kahlil Gibran, *The Wisdom of Kahlil Gibran*, edited by Andrew Dib Sherfan (London: Arrow Books, 1993), p. 149.

Chapter 1

1 Teresa (1515-1582), *Teresa of Avila: The Interior Castle* (translated by Kieran Kavanaugh), (Mahwah, NJ: Paulist Press, 1979), Ch. 2 v. 33.

2 It also happens that, in astrology, the various astrological signs are ascribed to various parts of the body. It's no surprise then to find that Pisces, the two fishes, is the sign attributed to the feet, linking the sole (fish) with the soul! There is a thread of ideas linking all the different meanings of similar sounding words. It goes like this:
   The sole fish's flat shape compares in its appearance to the bottom part of a shoe. Hence the origin of the word sole for this fish. There is also a connection with sea and sole found in the use of the word meaning the "spirit of a person". The old Germanic word *saiwalo,* from which the word soul was thought to originate, means the "soul of a person who was said to come from or belong to the sea," as the sea was thought to be the transitory stage of rest at birth or after death.
   From *saiwalo* also comes the word solo or sole, meaning alone (like the French soul/feminine *soule* and Latin *solus*).

The soul enters and leaves this world alone. Going into the sea is symbolically equivalent to plumbing the depths of our psyches, or to delve to the bottom of our emotional selves, hence the sole as the bottom of our physical body. This brings us back to the resemblance of the fish to the foot.

Etymology from: John Ayto, *Oxford School Dictionary of Word Origins* (Oxford: Oxford University Press, 2002) and:
Online Etymology Dictionary: http://www.etymonline.com

Chapter 2

1 Lao-tzu (604 BC - 531 BC), from *The Way of Lao-tzu*
2 Confucius (550 - 478BC) from *Analects*
3 Caroline Myss. *Daily Message of November 15, 2001* on her on her website: http://www.myss.com/myss/dailymsgarch.asp
4 William Shakespeare, *Hamlet*
5 John 1:1
6 Editors, *The Collector's Guide to Art and Artists in South Africa*, Preface, *(Capetown:* The SA Institute of Artists & Designers, 2003)
7 Socrates, (469 BC - 399 BC), from *"Apology,"* section 21, by Plato.

Chapter 4

1 Alison Motluk, *Asymetrical people make jealous lovers.*
New Scientist Print Edition, August 2002.
http://www.newscientist.com/article.ns?id=dn2698
"It seems that people who are more symmetrical are not only healthier, more fertile and perhaps even smarter - they are also more attractive." This led William Brown at Dalhousie University in Halifax, Nova Scotia, to wonder about jealousy. "If jealousy is a strategy to retain your mate, then the individual more likely to be philandered on is more likely to be jealous," he speculated. "And if people who are less symmetrical are less desirable, they are more likely to be cheated on."

Chapter 5

1 Socrates (469 BC - 399 BC). Plato. *The Last Days of Socrates*. Translated and with an introduction by Hugh Tredennick. (Middlesex, England: Penguin Books, 1961) pp. 71-2. In *Plato, Dialogues, Apology*. Socrates spoke these words to the jury in the court of Athens in the year 399 BCE (before the common era) after he had been found guilty of sedition and heresy. He chose death by the poison hemlock, rather than not being allowed to speak the truth. He told the court that he felt it was his responsibility, "... to let no day pass without discussing goodness and all the other subjects about which you hear me talking and examining both myself and others," and he felt that this activity, "is really the very best thing that a man (or women) can do, and that life without this sort of examination is not worth living..." Also information from: http://www.granpawayne.com/courses/EXAMLIFE.HTM

2 Carl Gustave Jung, "On the Psychology of the Transference," *The Practice of Psychotherapy: Essays on the Psychology of the Transference and other Subjects* (Collected Works Vol. 16). *CW 16*, (1966), p. 71.

3 William Blake, *On Another's Sorrow*.
   http://www.everypoet.com/archive/poetry/william_blake/william_bl ake_songs_of_innocence_on_anothers_sorrow.HTM_

SECTION TWO

1 From http://www.arthritis.org
2 Louise Hay, *Heal Your Body*, (Hay House Inc., Carlsbad, CA, 2001), p. 68.

List of Illustrations
All by Anthony Gadd

Bibliography

Ayto, John. *Oxford Dictionary of Word Origins.* (Oxford: Oxford University Press, 2002) and: *Online Etymology Dictionary:* http://www.etymonline.com

Bennett-Goteman, Tara. *Emotional Alchemy: How The Mind Can Heal The Heart.* London: Rider, 2003.

Campbell, Don. *The Mozart Effect: Tapping The Power of Music to Heal the Body, Strengthen the Mind, and Unlock the Creative Spirit.* London: Hodder Mobius, 1997.

Dethlefsen, Thorwald & Rudiger Dahlke, MD. *The Healing Power of Illness: Understanding What Your Symptoms Are Telling You.* Shaftesbury, Dorset, UK: Element Books. 1992

Evans, Philip. *The Family Medical Reference Book.* London: Time Warner Books, 2003.

Gribbin, John. *In Search of Schrodinger's Cat.* New York: Bantam Books, 1984.

Linn, Denise. *Pocketful of Dreams: The Mysterious World of Dreams Revealed.* Sydney, Australia: Triple Five Publishing, 1998.

Hay, Louise. *Heal Your Body.* Carlsbad, California: Hay House, 2001.

Hay, Louise. *You Can Heal Your Life.* Carlsbad, California: Hay House, 2001.

Judith, Anodea. *Eastern Body Western Mind: Psychology and the Chakra System as a Path to the Self.* Berkeley, California: Celestial Arts, 1996.

Myss, Caroline, Ph.D. *Anatomy of the Human Spirit: The Seven Stages of Power and Healing.* London: Bantam, 1997.

Sacks, Oliver. *An Anthropologist on Mars.* Random House Audio Publishing Group. Unabridged edition, 1995.

Sharma, Dr. R. (Editor). *The Element Family Encyclopedia of Health.* Shaftesbury, Dorset, UK: Element Books, 1998.

Stone, Joshua David, Ph.D. *Soul Psychology: How to Clear Negative Emotions and Spiritualize Your Life.* New York: Wellspring/Ballantine, 1999.

Stormer, Chris. *Language of the Feet: What Feet Can Tell You.* London: Headway, Hodder & Stoughton, 1999.

Thondup, Tulku. *The Healing Power of the Mind.* Boston: Shambhala, 1996.

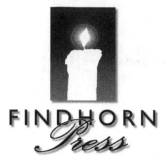

FINDHORN Press

Books, Card Sets,
CDs & DVDs
that inspire and uplift

For a complete catalogue,
please contact:

Findhorn Press Ltd
305a The Park, Findhorn
Forres IV36 3TE
Scotland, UK

Telephone
+44-(0)1309-690582
Fax
+44(0)1309-690036
eMail
info@findhornpress.com

or consult our catalogue online
(with secure order facility) on

www.findhornpress.com